the
abundance
of less

A Social Experiment of
Not Buying Anything New
for One Year

Marcy Pusey

Copyright © 2020 by Marcy Pusey
Published by Miramare Ponte Press
www.miramarepontepress.com

All rights reserved. This book is protected by copyright. No part of this book may be reproduced or transmitted in any form or by any means, including as photocopies or scanned-in or other electronic copies, or utilized by any information storage and retrieval system without written permission from the copyright owner.

Although the author and publisher have made every effort to ensure that the information in this book was correct at press time, the author and publisher do not assume and hereby disclaim any liability to any party for any loss, damage, or disruption caused by errors or omissions, whether such errors or omissions result from negligence, accident, or any other cause.

Adherence to all applicable laws and regulations, including international, federal, state and local governing professional licensing, business practices, advertising, and all other aspects of doing business in the US, Canada or any other jurisdiction is the sole responsibility of the reader and consumer.

Any internet address, company, or product information printed in this book are provided for informational purposes only; they do not constitute an endorsement or an approval by Marcy Pusey or Miramare Ponte Press of any of the products, services or opinions of the corporation or organization or individual. Marcy Pusey and Miramare Ponte Press bear no responsibility for the accuracy, legality or content of the external site or for that of subsequent links. Contact the external site for answers to questions regarding its content.

Neither the author nor the publisher assumes any responsibility or liability whatsoever on behalf of the consumer or reader of this material. Any perceived slight of any individual or organization is purely unintentional.

Neither the author nor the publisher can be held responsible for the use of the information provided within this book. Please always consult a trained professional before making any decision regarding treatment of yourself or others.

Printed in the United States of America.

Cover Design by 100Covers.com
Interior Design by FormattedBooks.com
Author Photo: Larisa Radcliffe
http://whitetree.photography

ISBN e-book: 978-1-948283-20-5
ISBN-13 Print: 978-1-948283-19-9
Library of Congress Control Number: 202091598

Get the
Abundance of Less Action Guide Free!

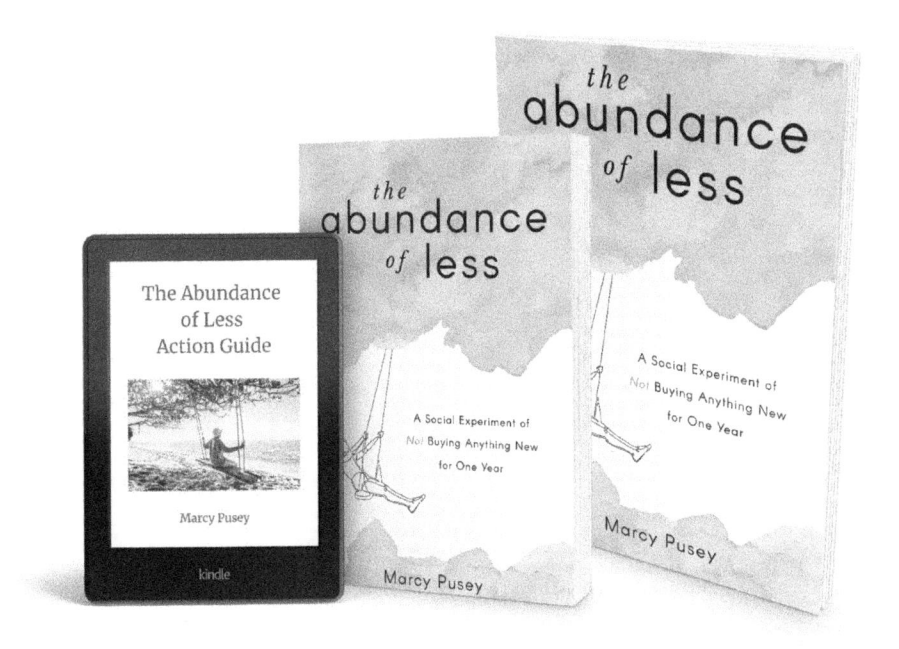

As a gift to help you get the most out of this book, we are giving you strategies, tips, and plans to help you execute your own year of living the abundance of less experience.

Download your free Action Guide at:

marcypusey.com/abundance-guide

Dedication

To everyone running in their own lane to make this world a better place. This is for you. Thank you.

Contents

Dedication v

Introduction ix
    Blog Post—January—A New Year Challenge xiv

Chapter 1: The Practicalities.. 1
    Blog Post—January—Why? 6

Chapter 2: Busting the Myths that Lead Us to Buy 7
    Blog Post—January—Paper Blessing....................................... 15

Chapter 3: Misplaced Priorities 17
    Blog Post—November—Fun Ways to Spend Your Money 22

Chapter 4: Hoarders and Extreme Collectors 25
    Blog Post—September—Little is Much 31

Chapter 5: It's Just an Upgrade.. 33
    Blog Post—June—Immersion Blender Freebie 40

Chapter 6: How Can I Change the World? Or Even Empty that Drawer? 43
    Blog Post—April—Birthday 47

Chapter 7: How to Start... 49
    Blog Post—January—The Blessing of Sharing........................ 59
    Blog Post—February—Simplify... 60

Chapter 8: Immediate Gratification 61
    Blog Post—January—Why Wait?... 71

Chapter 9: Living on Your Own Excess 73
    Blog Post—January—Moochers... 82

Chapter 10: Dealing with Embarrassment... 85
    Blog Post—January—Birthdays 91
    Blog Post—March—Celebrating Birthday Parties 92
    Blog post—April—Another Birthday..................................... 95

Chapter 11: Birthdays and Holidays 97
   Blog Post—December—Used Gift Exchange 102
   Blog Post—May—Resoluting in Disneyland 104
   Blog Post—December—A Second-Hand Christmas 106
   Blog Post—January 2010—Haiti and Me 108

Chapter 12: Travel 111
   Blog Post—February—Love Cruise and Bahamas 119
   Blog Post—January—New York- Fashion Capital of the World 121

Chapter 13: That Time We Failed 123
   Blog Post—October—Convenience Culture Pay Off 130
   Blog Post—August—Birthdays, Birthdays, & More Birthdays. 131

Chapter 14: Takeaway 135
   Blog Post—October—Celebrating A Cause
   (Other Than Myself) 139
   Blog Post—November—Candy Buy-Back 141
   Blog Post—December—What My Kids Think 143

Chapter 15: According to Our Kids 145
   Blog Post—November—Countdown is On! 147

Chapter 16: New Challenge 149
   Blog Post—January 2011—Last Day or First Day? 152

Chapter 17: Your Turn 155

About Marcy Pusey 157

Introduction

We have too much stuff.

So much stuff that we pay monthly to rent extra spaces just to keep it. We have shows like *Hoarders* and *Hoarding: Buried Alive*. Every nook and cranny and hole is filled with *stuff*.

All the while, companies continue to mass produce *more*. Ads convince us that we don't have enough, or that what we have is not good enough. That *we* aren't good enough without their latest product. The billboards scream discontentment at us. Our children plead and cry for one more *that*.

It's exhausting to think about, isn't it? You can't turn on the television, open a browser, a newspaper, magazine, or drive down the street without being confronted with the many things you still *need* to be whole. To be happy. To be worth something. To be *someone*.

There are so many books and blogs on the topic of simplifying because we've had enough! We want less! Studies are showing that less stuff equals less stress. I want less stress! But even the thought of doing something about all that mess—is stressful!

This is one of the reasons that, in 2010, my family of six decided to challenge ourselves to *not buy anything new for an entire year.*

Well, except things we couldn't (didn't want to) get used, like diapers, toilet paper, consumables like that.

We wanted to be one less family supporting the mass production of stuff. Were we going to make a dent in the national atmosphere? Was Walmart going to feel the pang of my absence?

Not likely.

Now Target—maybe.

Really, we wanted to see if it was possible. Could a family *really* live a whole year without purchasing new items? Is there really as much excess as we believe? This wouldn't necessarily reduce the amount of stuff currently in our home, *but* it would certainly reduce what comes in and how often.

No more impulse buys in the check-out line.

INTRODUCTION

No more last-minute runs to a 24-hour store to grab whatever we must have right then.

No more flashy Facebook Ad "buy now" clicks.

No more...*more*.

Well my friends, let me tell you—it *is* possible. A family like ours (and I'm sure like yours) can indeed live an entire year without buying anything new. I know because we did it. And not only did we do it, but our challenge the following year was to get rid of at least 50% of what we owned (we ended up getting rid of 90%, but that's a story for chapter 16).

And because of this challenge, I started one of the first ever Buy-and-Sell groups on Facebook. In fact, I didn't know of any others at all when I decided that I wanted more than Yahoo Groups and Craigslist could offer. I wanted my direct community involved, an easier-to-navigate forum, and easier access to finding used things and giving mine away. Facebook seemed like a great place to start, so I set it up and went to bed, not sure if anything would come of it. I mean, a community of buyers and sellers is only a community if people join.

In less than twelve hours, nearly 100 people had joined and were utilizing it. By the end of the week, over a thousand people were in the group and participating. Friends of mine around the country loved the idea and began to start Facebook groups in their local areas too. Facebook buy-and-sell groups are now international and a legit *thing*.

And we are just a normal ol' family. The items we had to find used were not luxury items to the average population. We weren't weeping over the Mercedes we couldn't buy or despairing over the brand of clothing we wouldn't get to wear anymore (though you can get these second-hand too!).

We have four children, two of whom we adopted through foster care (you can read more of *that* story in my book, *Reclaiming Hope: Overcoming the Challenges of Parenting Foster and Adopted Children*). My husband taught fifth grade in a low-income, low-performing school district in a decent-sized city. I worked part-time from home while raising our children. We lived on that one income and my partial bit. We were in a better financial situation than the one I grew up in, but still had to work hard to make ends meet. We strove to remain debt-free (once we reached that goal, woohoo!) which meant careful budgeting and vigilance.

We were really just your average family, living the average American-life, who suddenly were hit with this crazy idea—and we did it. And so can you.

> "There is enough in the world for everyone's need; there
> is not enough for everyone's greed." —Gandhi

While changing the world and the culture would be *awesome*, I'm all about changing it one family at a time, beginning with ours if we're a source of a problem that we recognize. And while I'm pretty sure the world didn't feel it the year we chose to only buy used, we were surprised by the many personal, familial, and community benefits that were born of it.

Many of the people I surveyed inside the Buy-and-Sell groups said things like this:

I can remember times when I picked up articles I'd bought from someone I didn't know, but after they invited me to stay a while, I ended up having some deep and meaningful conversations with them.

Our year of repurposing stuff also *purposed* friendships. We met people we might never have met. We had so many interesting conversations. We experienced God's provision for our needs in areas we normally rushed to meet ourselves. Our pace of life slowed down. We had opportunities to give our things away rather than hoard them, store them, or trash them.

There are so many benefits from simply choosing to live counter-culturally. It brought people together from all walks of life. It brought businesses together, families together, individuals together. One of the most fulfilling aspects was watching the community take the lead and make those benefits happen.

As Thakur S. Powdyel, a senior official in the Bhutanese Ministry of Education, said: "The goal of life should not be limited to production, consumption, more production and more consumption. There is no necessary relationship between the level of possession and the level of well-being."

Or as Mark Sagoff said in his essay in The Atlantic, "…Although we must satisfy basic needs, a good life is not one devoted to amassing material possessions; what we own comes to own us, keeping us from fulfilling commitments that give meaning to life, such as those to family, friends, and faith. The appreciation of nature also deepens our lives. As we consume more, however, we are more likely to transform the natural world, so that less of it will remain for us to appreciate."

This is what we experienced as a family, and which rippled into our community, and eventually in many communities. An increased level of well-being, more meaning in life, and a deeper appreciation for what we have. And we are not alone.

In one of the Buy-and-Sell groups, a person said, "Well I think to some extent it restored my faith in people. I'm probably a skeptical person, but this group has a decent amount of really nice folks."

Another said, "Cleaning out and minimizing equals a more organized and happy me; cash for my kids when they sell stuff equals their willingness to get rid of old stuff, too."

My point in writing this book is *not* to tell you that this is the one and only way to happiness, well-being, and a better planet. To say so would quickly make me a hypocrite because I'm sure *somewhere* in my life there are inconsistencies, due either to ignorance or apathy. We had a Prius once and felt great about it—until everyone started saying how much it affected the planet to *make* the car. My point is, we're not perfect and we don't live it all out perfectly.

But I *will* say that this challenge was life changing. In many ways, it extended beyond the year. It has shaped into a vision of community far beyond that of just getting a good deal and saving a buck. It's become about supporting one another, watching needs fill at just the right time, and being a part of something beautiful.

That's why I wrote this book. I want you to have the chance to taste this. You could choose to never leave your house (and thus never buy anything new) and be in every Buy-and-Sell group, but if you don't take the opportunity to engage the world around you, you'll totally miss the point. The world will be better, not just because we're doing our part to end mass-production (ha!) but because of the friendships that might come from it, the conversations that might inspire you, the smiles you might get when your junk is their gem.

I do promise that if you are willing to step into a year like the one that challenged us, and meet it face on for all it has to offer, you will experience more than you'd expect or imagine. In the next pages, I'll share how that year went: the successes, the failures, things learned, things experienced. You'll read about how my four kids flourished in this year (in spite of getting used gifts for Christmas and birthdays—yep!). You'll read about how our view and vision transformed along the way and how it forever impacted us in a way we'd *never* change.

Why spend another day wishing you had less stuff? Wishing you were less stressed by the clutter? Why waste another *minute* rushing from store to store to fill a hole that won't be filled with stuff anyway? Or spending money you might not really have on things you might not really need? Why not try a new way? Meet some new people along the way. You'll find we're a pretty snazzy bunch. She thinks so: "I love that I can *trust* this group and people keep their word. I give people my address and meet at my house. I know that no one will scam me here."

No one is going to scam you here, either. We're gonna tell it like it was, all the painful and all the blissful. All the mess and all the beauty. All the impatience and all the blessing. The frustrations and the surprises.

Join me on a journey of discovering how you can live well (and happily!) with what you have, contribute less to the mass-production and excess problem, and decrease stress and anxiety at the same time!

Blog Post—January—A New Year Challenge

I have often said to others (and myself): "How is it that companies make any money selling new stuff? There is *so much* used stuff out there; I don't think anyone really *needs* to buy anything new." Of course, I was speaking specifically of those living in the US—a country of excess. It seems to me that most new items purchased are either upgrades from already-owned items, bought new for convenience/warranty, or just because that's what we do.

One day I was pondering potential New Year's Resolutions and a thought popped into my mind. You know them. Those thoughts that show up that are *clearly* not yours. That was *this* thought: *What would it be like to go a year without buying anything new?* Hmmm...seemed plausible. I already buy a lot of things used or trade/swap on certain websites.

I began to think of all the things I'd need to buy before the first of January. Well, that didn't happen, but it probably should have! That said, my husband was quick to jump on the idea and here we are, a family of six, embarking on a journey of living off the excess of our nation. He found Hebrews 13:5 as a rock for our journey:

"Keep your lives free from the love of money and be content with what you have, because God has said, 'Never will I leave you; never will I forsake you.'"

There are a number of verses that could apply, but the idea of being content with what we have, not needing the newest model, and stretching ourselves to trust more deeply in God's provision is the flame igniting our excitement.

On that note, here are some exceptions to our "buy nothing new" rule. We will continue to buy groceries (I don't want your used broccoli. Actually, I'd love to live on your leftovers—bring 'em by *any time*.) We will exempt home necessities such as diapers, toothbrushes, toilet paper, shampoo. I *do not* want your used TP. Keep it. Flush it. We will also continue with service items, such as servicing our vehicles. I will have to continue to spend $35 per month for brand new clothing for my foster children until their adoptions are complete, as per the policy of the state of California. We are not allowed to buy them clothes at a thrift store/yard sale. I imagine this comes from past neglectful foster-parents who will always find ways to work around the system, while the rest of us rule-followers and kid-lovers deal with the restrictions. Sorry birth-kids...you're outta luck on this one.

Other than that, nothing new can be bought!

That said, here's how the first four days have gone. Jeremy was at Vons and almost grabbed a movie to buy, when my oldest son said, "Dad, aren't we *not* buying anything new?" Caught! Jeremy hadn't realized how easy it is to just grab something on a whim and go. It was also humbling to have our child remind him! Especially since we hadn't announced it to the family yet (yeah, our little eavesdropper).

In the first four days of this year, my sewing machine broke, my husband's Bible flew off the roof of our car, and a big drawer in my kitchen went kaput. We ran out of duct tape and lost our fireplace key.

I posted an ad on the Fresno Freecycle and got a bunch of duct tape AND masking tape free from a wonderful woman. Still waiting on the fireplace key.

Chapter 1

The Practicalities

I was driving along the streets of my city, setting my mind on what kind of challenge my family could tackle for 2010. I can't remember why I was even looking for a challenge, maybe it was something someone had said, or something I had read. Or maybe I was just looking to take my family on another one of my adventures.

The idea *fell* on me.

Don't buy anything new for one year.

What? I had never even considered this option. In the throes of diapers, laundry, meal planning and grocery shopping, parenting children of trauma through foster care, and trying to start my writing career...who had time to think about how to *not* get what we needed?

I had, however, found myself, in the previous weeks or months, noticing how much excess our country had, but I hadn't at all considered how I could change that. I was just your average mama (other than the taking in of strangers and mothering them) trying to keep the poop in the toilet or diaper, the food *on* the table, and joy in our house. We used plastic sandwich bags, microwaves, and disposable diapers. Okay, with my first, we used only cloth because somewhere in us, we are kind of free-spirit-hippies. But with my second (who ended up being 4th or 9th, depending on how you count the kids we've parented), we were *all in* with the disposable. I did not have time to rinse, clean, and repeat. I didn't even have time for regular showers. But I digress.

We were mostly your average people. And basically, while I've had lots of other crazy ideas, this particular one of not buying new things had never crossed my mind.

I immediately labeled the thought as divine inspiration, because *who would think of that?* Except maybe the activists out there who are always thinking about ways to impact world issues.

THE PRACTICALITIES

As soon as the idea landed, I knew it was the one. I also had a strong feeling my husband would be all in. And if I'm honest, I'll tell you that I thought it wouldn't be that hard. I'm not really a shopper. I don't love going to the mall or walking through a store and purchasing things. I don't even like window shopping. Growing up on welfare, window shopping just equaled seeing things I'd never be able to afford, so why torture myself? Shopping also meant spending money I didn't really want to spend, because what if I needed that money later? My parents had taught me to keep money close because it was very, very limited. So, I'll admit that I stepped into this decision with some arrogance, thinking that it wouldn't be that hard for someone who doesn't like shopping anyway.

Boy, was this an eye-opening, humbling experience. I didn't realize the extent to which I was happy to go replace something broken. Or how subject I was to impulse buys. That $5 DVD rack at Target? Why not? I mean, a movie for only $5! Seemed a small enough amount to not make a significant dent in our spending. Unless you grab every small deal you see—it adds up. I was about to realize how much this challenge would prove to be an actual challenge.

After talking it over with my all-in hubby, we determined some ground rules:

1. We would not buy anything new.

2. Exceptions to not buying anything new included:
    A) Consumables: diapers and toilet paper, namely. (Paper technically falls into this category, but if we *could* find it used or second hand, we did. Remind me to tell you a great story about paper later).
    B) Hand Made Items: This exception was spurred by a desire to turn our dollar toward local artists. Why support the companies who lie to us about our value and worth and acceptability in order to mass produce their product and live in luxury on my dollar and low self-esteem if I could *instead* send my dollar to another normal human trying to use his or her skill to get along in life? Whew! We weren't sure how often this opportunity would come up, but we wanted to keep it as a viable option instead of buying new from an established store.*[1]

C) Services: I value experiences over stuff. We wanted to maintain a lifestyle of doing life together, whether that was a road trip, a night out at a restaurant, or a trip to Disneyland. Naturally, we still had to live within a budget, but these experiences didn't fall under "new items."

3. We would embrace grace. I don't think we actually established that as a rule at the beginning…but it ended up we'd be needing it along the way. We had plenty of practice trying to live *grace* out. We made mistakes. We broke down. Slipped. Got back up and kept going. We acknowledged these moments to each other and to our readers as we blogged about our journey. We weren't out to establish a new law for ourselves and then beat each other up when we messed up. But we would make our best effort toward living out this challenge.

We began to feel excited about the challenge. We could be a part of something that makes a difference! We humans love to feel that our lives are lived for something greater. We have that in our hearts and home through our faith. But we also long to combine that faith with practical life activity to further a message of hope and peace and encouragement. Naive as we can be, we longed to see a better world for all. Realistic as we are, we knew we could only hope to make that change in our home first. As we learned more about the possible impact this idea could have, in our own small way, the more we were also encouraged to give it our all.

We began to see what David M. Walker meant when he said, "What we've got going are the elements of a perfect storm, a potent mix of ignorance, apathy, and inaction at all levels and in many sectors of American society. If we continue on our present course, a fiscal crisis is not a matter of if but when."[2]

Our own ignorance, apathy, and inaction had fed into this. While we often feel that our individual lives don't matter in the scheme of the grand national network, when *all* individuals believe this, we set the tone for the entire country. This requires some ownership of the national and global challenges caused by this mass production and over abundance.

There's a great song by one of my favorite bands, the Canadian group DownHere. In their song, *The Problem*, singers Jason Germain and Marc Martel weave us through all of the blame we like to cast: it's the government's fault, it's the devil's fault, it's *God's* fault, it's my neighbor's fault, before realizing, yeah, the world has problems and I'm one of those problems.[3]

It reminds me of the source of one of my favorite quotes by Gandhi: "We but mirror the world. All the tendencies present in the outer world are to be found in the world of our body. If we could change ourselves, the tendencies in the world would also change. As a man changes his own nature, so does the attitude of the world change towards him. This is the divine mystery supreme. A wonderful thing it is and the source of our happiness. We need not wait to see what others do."[4] It's from this quote that we get the often-quoted saying, "Be the change that you wish to see in the world."

Indeed, who am I to judge the state of the world if I am not doing *my* part to make it better? It's so easy to complain and grumble and judge and condemn, and never come up with a solution to offer. But how helpful is that? I try to practice following a complaint with a possible solution. This keeps me aware of the ways that I can contribute to change.

That being said, deciding to take on this challenge would come with its own form of pain. In a great article with detailed effects of our over-consumption on the earth, Chris Clugston says, "Terminating our addiction to excessive consumption would involve painful withdrawal symptoms: significant living standard disruptions—material living standard degradation and/or population level reductions, which we consider to be 'unacceptable.'"[5]

Earlier in his article, Clugston says, "Unfortunately, neither our addiction to excessive consumption nor our American way of life is sustainable… We, both individually and collectively, are the problem; we must be the solution…Excessive consumption is a self-induced societal disorder—a societal addiction. Every American is addicted to excessive consumption; we are all living beyond our means—most of us individually, all of us collectively, as the beneficiaries of the excesses perpetrated on our behalf by our political and economic representatives."[6]

Even if I personally am not living beyond my means, as a collective people, we are. What can I do to change Global Warming or drought, or famine, or disease in the world? I can change how *I* live.

I believe the idea to not purchase new things that day in my car was a call, not only to family adventure, but also to raise awareness in our own hearts to the ways we can "be the change" that we wish to see in the world, starting with our own wallets.

Now, in order to take our first step, we had to understand the myths. Just like anyone else, we had a list of beliefs that needed careful consideration as we moved forward. Were we going to save money? Would we lose all of our sources of happiness? Were we creating dependency in a land that prides itself on independence? In the next chapter, I'll cover the beliefs we realized were *myths* and the truths that exposed them, so we could tackle this challenge with integrity.

---

[1] I wish I could say this was all about stopping slave labor, and while I do care deeply about that horrible issue, I didn't know how to adequately make a difference there. But again, as individuals, we can do our part. Knowing the person I'm buying from, versus many unknown faces behind a brand, is a great way to begin taking steps toward ending slave and child labor in our own family spending.

[2] "Keeping America Great" presented by David M. Walker, Comptroller General of the United States, March 6, 2006, http://www.gao.gov/cghome/d061038cg.pdf accessed 10/30/16

[3] Jason Germaine and Marc Martel, The Problem, Ending is Beginning, Centricity Music, 2008, CD

[4] "The Collected Works of Mahatma Gandhi (Electronic Book), New Delhi, Publications Division Government of India, 1999, 98 volumes", Volume 13, pg 241 http://www.gandhiashramsevagram.org/gandhi-literature/mahatma-gandhi-collected-works-volume-13.pdf accessed 10/30/16.

[5] Chris Clugston, Excessive Consumption—America's Real Addiction, http://www.culturechange.org/cms/content/view/128/1/, accessed 10/30/16

[6] Chris Clugston, Excessive Consumption—America's Real Addiction, http://www.culturechange.org/cms/content/view/128/1/, accessed 10/30/16

Blog Post—January—Why?

I've been trying to put my finger on the *actual* reason I am doing this. I've had people ask, "Is it to save money?" No, though I hope that happens too. "Is it to be content with what you have?" Well, another hope, but also not the driving force. Finally, I figured it out.

I was looking in amazement at the eighty-one members who'd joined the Facebook group that I had spun from this idea, all within twenty-four hours of its start. I'm feeling so blessed by all of the conversations that are happening: the swapping, selling, taking, giving, sharing. And it hit me.

I am in love with community. I *love* to see the community of friends and family joining together to meet each other's needs. I love to see people helping each other out. I love to see someone find value in someone else's junk. It's such an awesome blessing! I am *not* buying anything new this year *so that* I can be a bigger part of a community that cares for one another. To give what I have and find what I need, and even those things that I just want. More importantly, I'm excited to see God meet our needs in a different way. We live in a country that has made it very easy for us to meet our own needs on our own time. That's not necessarily bad, but it is easy to forget the ultimate Gift-Giver.

I hope that this year ends filled with blessings all around as people rise up to share—a lesson we can't teach our children with words alone. Thank you for joining me and doing whatever you can to join the community of giving!

Chapter 2

Busting the Myths that Lead Us to Buy

I'm sure it comes as no surprise to you when I say that North Americans (and perhaps a few other Westernized countries) live in a state of constant excess. But why? How did we end up here?

I remember watching my mother-in-law pack up to move to Colombia. She pulled out fifteen-ish brand new toothbrushes. "These were on sale," she said, as she handed me a few. She explained that growing up in the Depression Era compelled her now, all of these years later, to grab a deal when she saw one and save for future hardships. I have found this to be common among that generation of people, the generation who'd lived on rations, lived on scarcity, lived with unmet needs (not just unmet wants). Their brains re-wired for survival. My mother-in-law made decent money. She didn't have to worry about whether or not she'd have future access to toothbrushes. But her experience growing up in the Depression had taught her to always be prepared, even in flourishing economies. Because you never know…

> To survive the Great Depression and make sure that whatever money was available was used for food, parents and families learned to make every available resource stretch – and they taught that technique to their children. Clothing was never thrown out. It was sewn or patched for re-use, and when it couldn't be worn any longer or handed down to another child, it was made into quilts or other fabric-based needs. Furniture, appliances and anything mechanical that couldn't be used any longer was saved. After all, you never know when you might

need a part from an old piece of machinery or furniture to stop-gap or fix another one. The "holding on to what you have" philosophy was one of safety. Nobody knew when the Depression would end or if it would get worse. The option to simply buy new things wasn't there. Most people wouldn't have survived if they hadn't learned to "hoard" possessions.[1]

But it did end.
Unfortunately, many of the children of this era taught the same scarcity mentality to their children, who taught it to their children, who taught it to their children. And even though we now live with extreme excess, many Americans have been raised to cling to everything "just in case."

An over-abundance of stuff isn't reserved for those of the Depression Era (or raised by those of the Depression Era). There are a number of other reasons we collect and buy and store. Mikael Cho, co-founder of oomph, says that we collect for a number of reasons. "Maybe you think you'll need to use it later, it has sentimental value, or you spent good money on it so you feel you need to keep the item, even if you haven't touched or used it in weeks, months, or years. You might be holding on to that book you bought a year ago that you swear you'll read or those killer pair of shoes that you'll bring out for just the right occasion."[2]

I think we also over-buy because of a few lies we believe. We've created a culture of convenience mentality, shifting our value from survival (Depression era) to status and self-importance (Abundance era). Because we have *so much* to choose from, we deserve to choose and own only the best. Unfortunately, the foundation of this thinking is based on a few myths. Let's bust 'em.

MYTH #1: Buying that next gadget will save me time in the long run.

TRUTH: Buying that next gadget will actually cost you time and energy.

According to the National Soap and Detergent Association (for real, there's actually a National Soap and Detergent Association) getting rid of clutter would eliminate forty percent of housework in the average home.[3] Buying that next little doohickey adds to the pile of things you'll need to dust, move, arrange, and clean around. Another study, compiled by the National Association of Professional Organizers (NAPO) in 2008, revealed that "twenty-seven percent of their survey participants said they feel disorganized at work. Of those, ninety-one percent said they would be more effective and efficient if their workspace was better organized. Twenty-eight percent said they would save over an hour per day and twenty-seven percent said they would save thirty-one to sixty minutes each day."[4] The cost of *more* even affects our work productivity and efficiency. The problem is not just in our homes.

MYTH #2: Buying that next thingy will save me loads of money.

TRUTH: Buying that next thingy will cost you thousands of dollars.

In a study by *Business Insider*, it was determined that nearly half of American households don't save any money, not intentionally month-to-month, nor in our many bargain buys. However, we *do* spend nearly $1.2 *trillion* annually on nonessential goods. Yeah, on stuff we don't even need. $1.2 trillion. Mark Whitehouse, of the *Wall Street Journal*, goes on to list things such as marshmallow peeps, hay, boats, jewelry, booze, gambling, and candy.[5] The study does *not* include super-fast cars or bigger-than-necessary houses, so the sum of $1.2 trillion is probably conservative. We then spend $8 billion buying home organization systems (stuff to organize our stuff).[6] And when your house runs out of space for all the stuff that organizes your stuff, you go rent a storage space, contributing to a $154 *billion* industry. We pay to store the stuff that stores our stuff so that we have room for more stuff. But you got the stuff at a great deal! Aren't you saving money?

No. No, you're not. I chuckle when I remember the times I've bought something on sale thinking, "Wow, I'm saving money!" only to realize that I had *spent* money I didn't need on something I hadn't thought I *needed* until I saw it there, gleaming on the discount shelf. I didn't save money—I'd spent money. And I'd added another "thing" to another shelf.

The COVID-19 pandemic of 2020 gave us a glimpse at what we really needed. Governments defined "essential" goods for us and only permitted their citizens to leave their homes to purchase these pre-defined items. In some countries, "essential" included beer and cigarettes (ironically, the very same things said countries heavily tax and make a lot of money from). In some countries, toilet paper was "essential" and in other countries, not. The restrictions on our purchases showed us what we actually *needed* in order to survive. It also made us realize how much *want* we took for granted. I'd like to believe it developed in us a sense of gratitude and awareness.

The next stat cracks me up, but it should be part of our cost-tally. The Harris Interactive Report apparently found that twenty-three percent of adults pay their bills late, incurring late fees—because they *lose the bills.* Some of us pay larger bills because we can't find the bills to pay them. Each month.

So, you're saving a few cents or dollars when you get the item on sale, but you're *still* spending money. And it's going to cost you to store that thing, whether it requires a shelf, a bin, or a drawer—or an additional storage unit. Or maybe you aren't paying for an extra storage unit, but you live in a house larger than what you need, because you like all of the "storage space." Instead of paying a monthly fee for storage to a storage company, you're paying it to the bank. Many of us are also now paying to store our digital stuff, paying clouds or services to hang on to it for us because our computer drives are too full. And we've taxed the free amount of space that Dropbox gives. So, we add another few bucks a month to store our files, our apps, our photos, our videos, and our work.

No, buying that thingy will *not* save you money.

MYTH #3: Buying that item will make me happy.

TRUTH: Buying that thing will make you stressed, frustrated, and angry.

An article in *Psychology Today* points out how "clutter bombards our minds with excessive stimuli (visual, olfactory, tactile), causing our senses to work overtime on stimuli that aren't necessary or important."[7] Excessive stuff prevents us from relaxing, physically and mentally. It constantly signals our brain that our work isn't done, so we don't trigger the pleasure center of our brain with accomplishment. It frustrates us when we can't find what we're looking for. It causes us to feel resentful toward the very things we purchased for our happiness. We use more emotional energy avoiding the guilt, the embarrassment, and the uneasiness that this causes us. We try to physically or mentally shove the stuff out of sight and out of mind because that seems "easier," but it's slowly killing us. Your home, which should be a haven, becomes a place in which you can't work or relax because of the constant visual stimuli. So, then we spend money to work outside of the home, go on vacations to get a "break" from the home, only to come back and find it all still there. And now we've spent more money (see Myth #2).

Stuff does not make us happy. It can't. Even as I write, I realize how much stuff I have again, even after getting rid of 90% of what we owned in 2012. Acquiring seems a little like breathing sometimes. When we moved to Germany to work at an International School, we had 44 boxes to our name. That was it. And most of those boxes were books and bedding and holiday decor. We didn't leave a storage shed of stuff behind in the States. We brought things that would help our young children maneuver the transition better, things that would make our new space in a foreign country feel a little more like home. All of that fit into our 44 boxes.

One day I came home, not too long after we'd arrived. Someone had dropped *bags* of toys on my porch. I imagine they were sure we missed all of the stuff we'd left behind. Or perhaps they were a gift-giver and wanted to bless our children with some "new" toys. Or maybe they'd been looking for a way to get rid of *their* excess stuff, and our porch seemed like the best way to do it, under the guise of "gifting" to a new family. Regardless, touches like this, in addition to trying to figure out what we needed and didn't need in this new land, has led, once again, to a house that feels too full for me. We love board games and keep buying them, and now have more than we can feasibly play. We have rooms full of toys that overflow their bins, clothes that overflow the hamper and drawers, books that overflow the shelves—too much.

MYTH #4: If I buy that doohickey, I will be more independent. True happiness and health come from self-reliance.

TRUTH: Happiness and health come from interdependence, not that doohickey.

Independence has been a high value in United States culture for some time. It's awarded us great freedoms, like *being* a nation free of monarchy and giving us rights to speech and religion. Autonomy is important. However, with time, the idea of independence has veered into a danger zone. People strive to be free from the control of others and their authority. We don't want to need anyone else to survive because, along the way, this has come to mean we are weak, ineffective, and worthless. The cream of the crop is capable, reliable, sufficient, and needs no one.

We see an ebb and flow of independence in the developmental and life stages of maturity, from dependent child, to independent adults, to dependent elder. But independence is not the final destination of a fully mature person. It is a *tool* through which someone can attain a level of freedom, a level of satisfaction, and yes, even happiness. But if you stay there, you remain under-developed. And under-developed people rarely experience ongoing true happiness or health.

As lone rangers, we become stunted. We can only grow and develop insofar as we have the awareness to do so. When we completely separate ourselves from the *other*, we lose the power and benefit of learning and growing from what they have to offer. The Bible says, "as iron sharpens iron, so one person sharpens another" (Proverbs 27:17). You will grow dull and weak if your goal is solely self-reliance.

I've found that a number of the things we buy promise us new freedoms and a sense of independence, but in reality, *cause* dependence. For example, the smart phone. It holds our calendar, freeing us up from carrying around a print calendar. It holds our emails, freeing up the space in our minds or on our desk for filing letters. It stores our photos, freeing up our ability to take as many as we'd like without clogging boxes in our basements. It holds access to unlimited sources of information, freeing our shelves of encyclopedias and our lives of the time spent reading them. Freedom, right? Independence! Self-reliance! You don't need anyone if you've got Siri. You've arrived.

Now, imagine five minutes with your phone missing. I've had this happen during meal-prep. I couldn't find a single print recipe from which to make our meal. I couldn't remember how to convert teaspoons into grams (which I need to do in Germany). Suddenly, my mind was totally blank, and I couldn't figure out how to put a meal together. Dependence. I had freed myself from Mom and Grandma being the source of my cooking heritage and turned to Google. Without Google, we live on packages of ramen and wurst. *Dependence.*

Without my phone, I feel the pain of having lost an arm. Or both arms. I no longer have anyone's phone number memorized. If I'm stranded on the side of the road and my phone battery has died, oh, you better believe I'm independent. But I'm not free. I'm *stuck*.

It doesn't matter what the *thing* is, we have to release the myth from our belief system that *stuff* makes us independent and healthy and operate from the truth that health and happiness come with *interdependence*. This is the fullness of maturity and human development. It's the awareness that I am more and can do more in connection with other humans. It's the discernment of what others can offer, discarding what's harmful and integrating what's wholesome.

In his book, *The Seven Habits of Highly Successful People*, Stephan Covey says about interdependence, "I have the opportunity to share myself deeply, meaningfully, with others, and I have access to the vast resources and potential of other human beings." Instead of saying, "I don't need anyone's help," interdependence says, "I bet I can do an even better job utilizing the gifts and resources of those around me." It's a growth-mindset, an appreciation for our own limitations and the infinite possibility of what is available to us when we acknowledge what others offer. When done right, it's harmony.

A family has the opportunity to model interdependence beautifully. Each person has a role and position. Each person is unique with various gifts, skills, and weaknesses. Acknowledging the differences and working together can create a peaceful, harmonious family life. Unfortunately, many people in families today operate from *independence* and self-centeredness. If each person in the home strives toward their own interest, the happiness-flow is disrupted. If each person is determined to need nothing from the other, you find a home of roommates, not family. James said, "What causes fights and quarrels among you? Don't they come from your desires that battle within you? You desire but do not have, so you kill. You covet but you cannot get what you want, so you quarrel and fight" (4:1). A family living interdependently with each other will have less tension in the home, less conflict, and greater life-satisfaction, which all leads to health and happiness.

Slowing down our rush to consume mass-produced items leads us into a place of *community*. Collaboration. Sharing what you have, utilizing what others offer. A world of people living interdependently, is a world promoting health and happiness. It's a circle. A world promoting health and happiness doesn't rely on the next bargain offer or discount ad. It finds health and wholeness in meeting the need of the other and in being met, as well.

As I write to bust these myths, please don't think I'm on any kind of self-made pedestal or that I've "arrived" at clutter-free heaven. This is a lifelong process. It gets easier, but it takes work to live on less and not buy more. With a good dose of re-prioritizing and re-evaluating what we want in life, the transition from too-much, too-often to just right and peaceful homes can happen. In the next chapter, we'll take a look at the how priorities and values inform our purchase habits *and* our health and happiness.

---

[1] "Did Clutter and Hoarding Start with the Depression Generation?" by Postconsumers Content Team May 3, 2013, https://www.postconsumers.com/2013/05/03/depression-era-hoarders/, accessed 10/29/16

[2] How Clutter Affects Your Brain (and What You Can Do About It) Mikael Cho, Lifehacker, lifehacker.com/how-clutter-affects-your-brain-and-what-you-can-do-abo-662647035, accessed 10/29/16

[3] BecomingMinimalist.com by Joshua Becker, http://www.becomingminimalist.com/the-statistics-of-clutter/, accessed 10/29/16

[4] BecomingMinimalist.com by Joshua Becker, http://www.becomingminimalist.com/the-statistics-of-clutter/, accessed 10/29/16

[5] Number of the Week: Americans Buy More Stuff They Don't Need by Mark Whitehouse, April 23, 2011, http://blogs.wsj.com/economics/2011/04/23/number-of-the-week-americans-buy-more-stuff-they-dont-need/, accessed 10/29/2016

[6] Clutter Stats by Joshua Becker, http://www.becomingminimalist.com/clutter-stats/, accessed 10/29/16

[7] Why Mess Causes Stress: 8 Reasons, 8 Remedies by Sherrie Bourg Carter Psy.D, Psychology Today https://www.psychologytoday.com/blog/high-octane-women/201203/why-mess-causes-stress-8-reasons-8-remedies, accessed 10/29/16

Blog Post—January—Paper Blessing

Normally "paper blessings" might imply something flimsy, semi-transparent, or lightweight. Not today.

I made a request on Freecycle and the LivingHebrews135 Facebook group for computer paper. Scrap, half used, or extra. Not something that would cost or be unethical (i.e., I don't want your work paper if you have to steal it from work. Just your excess.)

I was immediately met with a dilemma to my request; it caused me to really think about what is "okay" to buy new and what isn't. Before I finished deciding, the offers were coming in.

Two separate women quickly responded to my requests, full of encouragement and appreciation for our resolution. Both had paper that was excess, and both felt that Freecycle was exactly the place to make such a request (I asked their opinions).

Well, the first woman ended up being someone with whom I'd shared some of our baby things. When it was *she* who showed up at my door, I was blessed all over again. I can only imagine how good it felt for her to *return* a favor and for me to be the recipient of what she now had to offer. I took note of God's detail.

The next woman owns Secondhand Rose. This is a thrift store that opened last summer on Shaw and Armstrong. Maybe that sounds way out there, but it's really not. She has a great little store, but the "catch" is that a portion of her profits goes to military families. She has a heart for helping people and often gives things from her store to people on Freecycle asking for it. She embroiders, sews, makes beautiful dolls and baby things, as well as sells second-hand items. She'd found a big box of 8 1/2 by 14 paper on the side of the road. No one has wanted to buy it from her store, and she saw my request. I went to her store to get paper and left with a total blessing. Visit her store if you can! You don't just buy used, but you help the families of our soldiers when you do!

Then today a dear woman from church asked if I was still needing paper. I said, "Sure!" She brought me two brand new reams that she had extra and said, "My husband mentioned you might have some legal sized paper, that's what he uses if you don't need it." Well, PRAISE THE LORD! Now I don't have to cut the last couple inches off. I get to give it to someone who needs it *and* in return get more 8 1/2 by 11 paper!

Ya know, on any other day or year, I would have run to Walmart and just bought some paper. I would have missed all of these blessings—a favor returned, a conversation with a servant, and the opportunity to give what I have. I certainly didn't expect paper to be so rewarding!

This is all causing me to wonder—how many times has my need for immediate gratification robbed God of a blessing for me? How many wonderful people have I missed meeting? Or ministries have I missed contributing to? Or robbed others of blessings? Or myself been robbed?

I hope that the end of this year will find me a more patient person for the things I think I need.

And in return, may I become a less hurried and more intentional person.

Wouldn't it be so cool if life wasn't actually about the end goal? But instead about the journey of getting to it?

Chapter 3

Misplaced Priorities

Once we're able to get some of the lies we've believed out of the way, we can begin to refocus on what's *true* and what's *helpful*. Have you ever heard of the T.H.I.N.K. acronym, used as a filter before speaking? Is it True? Is it Helpful? Is it Inspiring? Is it Necessary? Is it Kind? Not only should these questions guide how we speak to others, but they should guide how we speak *to ourselves*. These are great questions we should also ask ourselves before purchasing something *at all*, let alone brand new. Is what I believe about this item true? Is this item helpful? Does it inspire me? Is it necessary? Is it a kindness to purchase this item, for myself *and* for others?

Because we've had no real guide, only the loud voices of media and marketers, we've lost our way with priorities.

In the land of freedom, we've become slaves to our own happiness.

Except, it turns out, that happiness isn't a very great master.

According to *Psychology Today*, Americans spend more money on shoes, jewelry, and watches ($100 billion) than on higher education.[1]

In the book, *Affluenza: The All-Consuming Epidemic*, the authors claim that thirty percent of Americans buy Christmas presents for their pets. And that shopping malls outnumber high schools in America.[2]

Our right to the pursuit of happiness has led us to think that we deserve happiness at any cost, and so we are trying it all. If we think for a minute that something might make us happy, we grab it. And when it doesn't make us happy, it sits on a shelf and we grab the next thing. The "thing" can be relationships, jobs, food, gadgets, college degrees—anything that we can have. The thing is, they don't normally bring us the happiness they promise (as covered in Chapter 2). Which is why we keep striving to find that *thing*, that right thing, that right job position or salary or friend or lover or pet or scrapbook paper or car or device or (fill in the blank) that will finally fulfill its promise.

Happiness is not bad. In fact, I believe we are designed to seek it. But we've gotten what *brings* happiness all wrong. And in doing so, we've begun to kill the pleasure-centers of our brain, making the feeling of happiness, contentment, satisfaction, and joy that much harder to access.[3] In our pursuit of happiness, we've often become discouraged, disillusioned, and given up, numbing our brains and hearts away to push down the fact that nothing can make us happy. In homes full to the brim of everything that was supposed to.

"We are possessed by our possessions; they are often harder to get rid of than to acquire…Well-being depends upon health, *membership in a community in which one feels secure*, friends, faith, family, love, and virtues that money cannot buy…"[4] (emphasis mine).

And really, here's my bias. I don't value shoes over higher education. There, I said it. I don't value animals over hungry people (even though I'm an animal-lover). Peter G Stromberg, author of *Psychology Today*, points out that "arguments about over-consumption are in fact thinly-disguised discussions about values and politics. And since we are all consumers, these discussions always come down to assertions by one person that he or she is buying the right stuff and other people are buying the wrong stuff." It's true. The more I speak about consumption and excess and our part, the more I realize how the conversation veers toward values.

It's easy to determine for *another* person what is clutter, excess, or an appropriate buy. That is not my purpose here. Instead, I believe that our nation produces far too much stuff, and in that excess, we lose sight of what matters. We also perpetuate the lies that we will be happier, financially free, and have more time on our hands. We, as a nation, are stuck in a crazy-cycle and need help getting out of it. We want happiness and satisfaction, but we keep bringing on stress, strife, and emptiness instead. Maybe this is why we are seeing, in our American society, people who over-react, are explosive, and entitled. Because we don't have the emotional space for *any* disturbance in the force.

This is evidence that maybe some values are more beneficial for a person or a society than others. Maybe valuing the toll our waste takes on the earth over having access to free plastic shopping bags at the checkout is more beneficial for each of us, even though the values differ. Our values can be based on ignorance, misperception, or myths. The right information can help us shift our values. For example, if you desire a stress-free life, and you learn that cats cause you stress, you'll have a decision to make. You can change your stress-free living value *or* get a new pet.

Some of us just haven't known another way.

Hence the great number of books, blogs, articles, and videos surrounding the themes of margin, Sabbath, sabbatical, rest, and LESS. We are so inundated that we can't take it anymore. We have to do something differently. We need less.

I don't know if you're like me, but sometimes just the *thought* of stepping into a cluttered room or brain-space is enough to send me to my bed for a nap. It's exhausting to consider, let alone take an actual step toward. But this just prolongs the pain. We must learn new ways.

I mean, we'll *have* to learn things. Not all of the Depression-era skills were bad. We can leave some in the past, but some belong in our present, like how to re-use what we have. How to recycle. Upcycle. Let's sew a hole shut instead of rushing off to Target and simply buying a new shirt. Did you know that the average American home has over 300,000 items in it?[5] And it's still not enough. The average American woman owns an outfit for every day of the month. In 1930, women owned, on average, nine outfits. Nine.[6] What do we do with all of these clothes? Well, according to a Huffington Post article, we throw a bunch of it away. On average, Americans throw away sixty-five pounds of clothing, per person, each year.[7]

I had the deep privilege of working with refugees on Lesvos in Greece in 2016, at the height of all of the Syrian asylum-seekers making their way in inflatable rafts from Turkey to Greece. I did a number of things, including give warm clothing and hot food to sea-drenched dreamers-of-a-new-life. But I also *sorted* whole warehouses of donated clothing in anticipation of the refugees who'd need a new start. You would not *believe* the amount of clothing that had been donated for this cause. What struck me wasn't so much how generous people had been in their donations (though they had been) but how *much* people had to give, and still remain sufficiently clothed themselves (I assume). Groups of volunteers cycled through the warehouses for hours at a time, all day, and hardly made a dent in the offerings. It was incredible!

But the other reason sorters were required was because a good chunk of the donated clothing was just straight *junk*. People, do *not* donate something you wouldn't yourself wear because of stains or holes. Do not send *dirty* clothes. It was almost as if people were aware of the need to Spring Clean and expel their excess, but instead of simply throwing some of what they owned in the trash where it belonged, they threw it in a donation bin, where fundraised money shipped it across the world, stored it in warehouses, only to be dumped in the trash bins of an island already overwhelmed with trash. Our own resistance to *throwing things away* simply transferred the problem of one person's closet to the dump yard of a country struggling to care for its own while suddenly being inundated with penniless immigrants.

Getting our priorities straight is going to take some work. It's also going to take some humility. We will have to acknowledge that we've been going about some things in the wrong way. In a way that is causing us harm. A way that is causing our children and our neighbors and the world harm. We are going to have to recognize and own that we've been doing life in a crazy-cycle sort of way—doing the same thing over and over but expecting that somehow *this time* it will be different. *This* item will finally bring long-term satisfaction.

We also have to acknowledge that we've been lied to. Billions of dollars are spent by companies to convince us that what we have isn't enough. That our social status isn't high enough, our clothing isn't the right brand, our car doesn't have enough cylinders, to be truly happy. And they're lying.

Because happiness is far less about *stuff* and far more about our sense of well-being.

Now that we've considered ways that our priorities influence our spending, we'll take a look at what happens when well-being gets wrapped up excessive consumption and the impact on those individuals and their families.

---

[1] Do Americans Consume Too Much by Peter G Stromberg, PhD., https://www.psychologytoday.com/blog/sex-drugs-and-boredom/201207/do-americans-consume-too-much accessed 10/29/16

[2] Affluenza: The All-Consuming Epidemic by John deGraff, David Want, and Thomas Naylor. September 1, 2005. Page 13

[3] Hart, A. D. (2007). Thrilled to death: How the Endless Pursuit of Pleasure is Leaving us Numb. Nashville: Thomas Nelson

[4] Consumption: Theory and Issues in the study of Consumption, edited by Daniel Miller, pg 450

[5] For Many People, Gathering Possessions is Just the Stuff of Life, by Mary MacVean, March 21, 2014, http://articles.latimes.com/2014/mar/21/health/la-he-keeping-stuff-20140322, accessed 10/29/16

6   Forbes, http://www.forbes.com/forbes/welcome/?toURL=http://www.forbes.com/sites/emmajohnson/2015/01/15/the-real-cost-of-your-shopping-habits/&refURL=&referrer=, accessed 10/29/16

7   Closet Cast-Offs Clogging Landfills by Mattias Wallander, The Huffington Post, May 25, 2011, http://www.huffingtonpost.com/mattias-wallander/closet-cast-offs-clogging_b_554400.html, accessed 10/29/16

Blog Post—November—Fun Ways to Spend Your Money

I'm going to offer a newfound (by my family, anyway) activity that gives your money to a number of great causes: a charity, your physical and mental health, family bonding!

We have discovered family races or walks that support a cause and encourage the idea among my family that fitness is "fun" even if *you* don't think so. I knew that I couldn't teach my children something that I wasn't walking. Hence, in order to prove to them that fitness was indeed fun (which I didn't personally believe), I began to do it... in front of them. Jogging, family walks, family bike rides, workout videos, whatever! I have the cutest video of my two-year-old doing the exercises he always saw me doing and *loving* it! What a treasure!

We live in such an obese society that on my list of "Things I Want for My Kids" I have one, in love with Jesus and two, healthy. They have seen me lose twenty-five pounds and a couple dress sizes in the last year as I've raced to prove to them how much fun fitness is!

That said, I joined an amazing team of people who committed to running a half marathon and raising sponsors (like a jog-a-thon) in order to bring awareness and support to my friends, the Gilmores. They are moving to Haiti in January (Lord willing) in order to "live the need" among the Haitians in all of their current plights. It's one thing to hear about the need from friends...and a whole other thing to commit to understanding it through experiencing it. This is their goal.

This commitment (which I made in total ignorance—13.1 miles is a lot of miles to run!) has kicked me into many of the smaller races around my town. I have found that *many* of them raise money for great causes and are just plain fun! We did Feet for Families to raise money for Adoption and Foster Care. That was a simple 3.1-mile race (or a two-mile walk) and we got breakfast and all sorts of freebies! We also did a Walk for Huntington's Disease—two miles easy. At this one, my friend Dorina and I won a free Me-n-Eds pizza and a t-shirt for playing ping-pong with a snorkel flipper and shaking a ping pong ball out of a tissue box...attached to my bootie. AND, lastly, we've just signed up for the Turkey Trot, a fun tradition for many families on Thanksgiving Day. Why not walk off all your meal before you eat it? Plus, "free" socks for the first 1200 to sign up!

All of these family walks and events were about $12 or less and supported causes we connected to. Plus, our family was able to spend the day doing something fun, for a common cause (not our *own* cause) and enjoying some physical activity. Not bad!

I just completed the half marathon yesterday. That was hard work! But I love what it has done for my body and my mind. I know that I can keep up with my kids. I *feel* better about myself. And my kids are my greatest (and cutest) cheerleaders!

So, go at it! Use your money in a way that builds your family in so many worthwhile ways! Not on the next video game, movie, TV show, or "hottest" toy off the shelf! All of that will burn away, but the time you spend together (supporting others) can never be undone!

Chapter 4

Hoarders and Extreme Collectors

I'm sure you look at that chapter title and think, "That's not me. I don't hoard. And I'm not an *extreme* collector. That's for reality TV." And you're probably right. But I think we all have something to learn from, and fear, when looking at the truly painful and disordered life of a hoarder or extreme collector.

The DSM-5[1] has listed Hoarding as an actual diagnosable and treatable disorder.[2] Studies show that people who hoard make up two to five percent of the American population. That's somewhere between six and sixteen *million* people. See, two and five percent don't sound like much—until it's millions of people. There's even an entire organization dedicated to the children of hoarders. Here's the thing that might sit between *you* and a person who hoards: Ego Dystonic. The person finds the behavior disturbing but feels unable to stop the behavior. Or maybe this doesn't sit between you and that person and you've just realized you *are* that person. Don't worry, there are at least six million other people who get it.

The DSM-5 says about Hoarding:

> Hoarding disorder is characterized by the persistent difficulty discarding or parting with possessions, regardless of the value others may attribute to these possessions. The behavior usually has harmful effects—emotional, physical, social, financial, and even legal—for the person suffering from the disorder and family members. For individuals who hoard, the quantity of their collected items sets them apart from people with normal collecting behaviors. They accumulate a large number of possessions that often

fill up or clutter active living areas of the home or workplace to the extent that their intended use is no longer possible. Symptoms of the disorder cause clinically significant distress or impairment in social, occupational or other important areas of functioning including maintaining an environment for self and/or others. While some people who hoard may not be particularly distressed by their behavior, their behavior can be distressing to other people, such as family members or landlords.[3]

Maybe you're feeling a little better now.

The thing about people who have a compulsion to collect and keep is that the symptoms are really hard to cover up. For this reason, people diagnosed with Hoarding have a *huge* impact on the people living with them. This piles on the guilt and shame and frustration of not being able to stop, which is often taken out on housemates in anger.

This is also why sites like childrenofhoarders.com exist. The site lists many of the challenges of living with a person who hoards. There is no functional living space, which leads to buying storage. After a short time, however, the storage is full and overflowing and the home returns to a place with no functional living space. No place to sit, no place to eat, no place to walk.

The effect on children of hoarders is greater than just walking space (although dangerous walkways is a valid concern, all by itself). Families of hoarders often live with mildew and fungus. Because there is so little room with all of the stuff, if something spills, or a dog pees, or dust falls (ahem), it is very difficult (if not impossible) to clean, leading to dust mites, mildew, mold, and fungus in the home. It can also lead to insect and rodent infestations. These all lead to poor health conditions, like asthma, and medical expenses. It's also a huge concern in the event of a fire.

Children and family members also deal with the emotional burden of living with a parent who hoards. They are often too embarrassed to invite anyone over to the house, and panic if someone wants to come over or shows up unexpectedly. Some situations become even more dire, and a concerned neighbor or friend calls Child Protective Services. In this case, the hoarding behavior can actually lead to the removal of children from the home, which has long-lasting, detrimental effects for all. Some families are aware of this, creating a culture of secrecy, as with any addiction. Children learn to keep the family secret so that they don't lose their home and their parents. What a burden for a child to carry! The alternative is that the child continues to live in the chaotic, dangerous home space. Both options are damaging.

An article in *Psychiatric Times* said about children of hoarders, "A person's value becomes secondary to a 'good deal.' As family members struggle through, hoarders often feel criticized, rejected, and shunned, and they turn to objects for safety, success, and the fulfillment of many misguided beliefs or values. Hoarders cannot see that their behavior subjugates the entire family to a life that is permanently altered."[4]

And they can be really nice people! But they live under a compulsion to collect that makes everything else secondary, including their relationships. In fact, if a family member were to try to *clean* or secretly get rid of things…bad. The result is fighting, arguments, fractured relationship, and the stuff stays. The hoarder just wants everyone to mind their own business because "it's not that big of a deal."

After seeing all of that, it's easy to feel really good about my own clutter. I mean, at least it's not like *that*, right? I can see my floor (mostly). I can dust (if I want to). I only have one junk drawer in the kitchen. My clothes fit in the closet.

This doesn't give us permission, in my opinion, to continue living in excess, even if it's *less* excess than someone else. Excess is still excess, and it still affects us. It affects you. It affects your children. Our own distorted view of *stuff* and its importance is the inheritance of our kiddos. But it doesn't have to be. We can work toward a healthier understanding of *things*.

Because they *do* matter.

We collect things because we hear an underlying message when we own that thing.

We might hear, "You're someone special. Way more special than *that* guy who can't afford this. He'll probably think so too."

Or, "*Now* you're beautiful."

Or, "I don't have to be afraid of the future. See? I can provide for myself."

Sometimes it brings us a sense of connection to someone we've loved and lost, or someone who matters to us. Things can evoke memories or re-inspire feelings from a different time. According to Randy Frost, PhD, Professor of Psychology at Smith College in Northampton, Massachusetts, "Emotional/sentimental attachment is a central motive for hoarding. The person anthropomorphizes the possession, believing that he or she will 'hurt the feelings' of the possession by discarding it. Other motives concern the use of possessions ('you never know when it can come in handy') or worry about information or memory loss ('if I discard this, I will forget its content or the event it represents')."[5]

I *know* you can relate to some of that. In fact, I can remember clearly, as a child, being positive that my stuffed animals could have hurt feelings. I was careful not to say which one was my favorite in front of them. (The hit movie *Toy Story* only fanned that flame for children, didn't it?) I know I personally feel a nudge to buy something I *might* need in the future. I've had a bag of fabric sitting in my basement for four years. Ouch. It pains me to write that. *Four years*. Because I have a plan to use it on an art project. Really. And if I think about it, I *might* have a few other things lying around waiting for an art project. (Ironically, the fabric was finally used to make facial masks in the Covid-19 Pandemic. See? I knew I would need it someday.)

But why? What drives me to that? Is it a fear that it won't still be accessible to me when I want it? That's the case with the fabric. I was in California where I could go to Jo-Ann's and buy awesome fabric for way less than I could get it in Europe. So, I did. Four years later…

Or is it because I'm afraid the sale will never come back again? Or that someday I'll have a need and won't be able to meet it if I haven't tucked away this thing?

"The notion that things don't matter is rubbish, the experts say. They matter for many reasons: keeping up with the Joneses, recalling departed loved ones, even objective value—like the 17th century Dutch painting that is among many objects of desire in Donna Tartt's 'The Goldfinch.' Our things can give us a sense of security, connection to the past, to the people we love."[6]

We can all find a reason to buy something. And buy it again. Or buy its upgrade. Or hang on to something that we never use. Or that we keep for four years sitting on the basement floor. It's not beyond us to begin to hoard and collect, even if we don't full on qualify for the DSM-5 diagnosis.

Understanding what drives us to consume is a huge part of how we'll ever get a handle on our consumption.

Personally, I have to insert a moment of self-awareness between an item and the checkout line. Do I really need this? What do I believe this item will do for me? What does this item communicate to me about myself? Is there a lie behind why I believe I should buy this item? Do I *love* it? What is the cost? (And I don't just mean financial). Does it already have a place in my house? And what can *go* if I bring this *in*? These questions often lead me to return an item to the shelf. Boom. Score for team consume-less-and-save-the-world-or-at-least-my-wallet.

Try this the next time you're scrolling on Amazon, hovering over that sweet "buy now" button, or walking the aisles of a store that seems to say, "It's okay, you're home now. We love you. Take anything you'd like (but leave your credit card number behind)." Pause and T.H.I.N.K. about it. Then ask yourself these same questions:

Do I really need this?

What do I believe this item will do for me?

What does this item communicate to me about myself?

Is there a lie behind why I believe I should buy this item?

Do I love it?

What is the cost (financial and otherwise)?

If it's an impulse buy, challenge yourself to wait twenty-four hours to reflect on the questions. If they all turn out legit, then it will be *worth* getting back in the car and finding that treasured, must-have, passed-the-test item.

If it's already gone? Well, consider yourself having saved some money! Your life went on without the item through today, it will continue after today as well. *Everything will be okay.*

At least, that's what I tell myself when I feel the panic rise in my chest. The heat of *but I wanted it! And it's not here! Who will I be now?* Whoops. Maybe it hadn't passed the test after all.

Hoarding isn't the only way to get caught up in over-consumption. In the next chapter, we'll take a look at a sneaky way marketers get into our wallets and how to stop them!

---

[1] American Psychiatric Association. (2013). Anxiety Disorders. In Diagnostic and statistical manual of mental disorders (5th ed.) https://doi.org/10.1176/appi.books.9780890425596.dsm05

[2] http://www.dsm5.org/Documents/Obsessive%20Compulsive%20Disorders%20Fact%20Sheet.pdf accessed 10/29/16

[3] http://www.dsm5.org/Documents/Obsessive%20Compulsive%20Disorders%20Fact%20Sheet.pdf accessed 10/29/16

[4] The Hidden Lives of Children of Hoarders by Suzanne A. Chabaud, PhD., Psychiatric Times, Nov 10, 2011, http://www.psychiatrictimes.com/obsessive-compulsive-disorder/hidden-lives-children-hoarders, accessed 10/29/16
[5] Managing Hoarding Disorder by Batya Swift Yasgur, July 27, 2015, accessed 10/29/16
[6] For Many People, Gathering Possessions is Just the Stuff of Life, by Mary MacVean, March 21, 2014, http://articles.latimes.com/2014/mar/21/health/la-he-keeping-stuff-20140322, accessed 10/29/16

Blog Post—September—Little is Much

There's a really great song by the amazing band DownHere called *Little Is Much*. Buy it.

It's so true though. I was in my garage yesterday. I have a bin beside my door for shoes. I have another bin beside my laundry for rags and towels. Actually, I *had* bins in these two places.

The rules were: Only shoes in the bin. No clothes in the towel bin.

But what do I find every time? Socks in the shoe bin and clothes in the towel bin. AH! So, what did I do? I tossed the bins! Put in a nice shelf for the shoes and said, "Throw the towels in the washing machine." Little is much. Little is *more*.

I've also done this in my kids' rooms. It seemed that if there was a cranny to shove a piece of trash or soiled clothing—they stashed it! So, I took it all out. They have a bed and a desk. No dresser. No bookshelf. Clothes all get hung. They have organizational bins in their closet for school, art, and personal. That's it. And it's amazing how much cleaner a room can be with less stuff in it.

I've even read studies lately stating that with all our technology we are producing *less*. And that the more *stuff* a person has around them, the higher their stress levels. On a personal level, this seems so true. Before Facebook my house was a lot cleaner! Or, maybe that was before *kids*! They both kind of kicked off about the same time, so I'm not really sure who the culprit is!

Anyway, as we try to live on the excess of our nation and to support our friends as homemakers and local businesses, we are also finding that getting rid of stuff is so freeing.

Even my three-year-old gets it. His sister tried to give him a new cool bracelet. He checked it out, said it was "cool" and gave it back.

She said, "No, it's yours." He said, "I don't need it." She tried to convince him that it was still his, but he was adamant: He didn't need it.

May I be as quick to get rid of the things I don't need and thus free myself of more stress and perhaps even become more productive! Lessons from a three-year-old.

Chapter 5

It's Just an Upgrade

There's the kind of excessive consumption that buys fifteen toothbrushes that are on sale, and the kind that keeps buying the same thing that we already have, just because a newer model is available. Every marketing team has a master of upsells and upgrades. Why? Companies really want to keep taking your money, and if you're satisfied with what you already have, then you won't buy anything else from them. So they sell you the item that promises you happiness, security, and popularity, only to tell you a few months later that it's no longer good enough—but don't worry, they now have *the* item that will bring you happiness, security, and popularity. And also, it's really cool. It does this thing that your last purchase can't do. A thing that you never knew you needed done for you before, but now it all seems so clear, your life has never been all that it could be because none of your possessions could do that thing. But now it's available.

There's a new pile in many homes. It's an outdated device pile. It's a pile that shows our incredible wealth, and perhaps stupidity. How many homes have multiple old phones? We can't find anyone to take them off our hands because they are so old, like, at least five months old. (However, I *am* that person who will buy your "old" phone because I'm too cheap to buy a new one.) I've even encountered the problem with teenagers having too many phones, because for some reason, they keep giving them to one of *my* children (the one least responsible with devices, naturally). Really? We have that much technology sitting around that we can give it away?

It's just an upgrade, right?

An upgrade every couple of years, or when your contract offers you one for free—I get that. I *don't get* the pile of growing junk in our homes because we keep buying the newer, better, more satisfying lie…I mean, model.

WHY?

I believe, as I've said in other chapters, that even upgrades speak something to our emotional sense of wellbeing. Starbucks, specifically, is really good at this. Starbucks' Secret of Success Number Three,' according to Michael Chibba, international business and development expert, is their ability to create the Starbucks Experience.[1] Depending on where you are in the world, Starbucks has created an experience for you, based on cultural values. For example, if you're in the U.S., the experience will involve incredible customer service and personalization. If you're in Asia, your experience will elevate your sense of prestige or status to be drinking Starbucks. If you're in Europe, that experience will involve knowing that your coffee is organic and a local brand. Of course, there are similarities in the Starbucks Experience across nations, for example, the sense of "home" when you enter the carefully decorated cafés. The feeling that somehow, even though you're a student or a member of the working class, you are "cool" too, because you are a Starbucks customer. Your Starbucks Experience is also going to include, no matter where you are, efficiency, sped-up service, free high-speed wi-fi, and custom-made drinks.

Why are you willing to pay more for a coffee? Some might beg to say because the coffee is actually better, but the majority (in my experience) say that it's for the experience. It's for the café atmosphere with free Internet and drinks with your name on the cup. This is successful marketing and it's everywhere.

I used to work in a movie theater (which I loved). We were taught to upsell the customer. "You know, you can get a large popcorn for only $1 more, and it's refillable." Same with the drinks. The managers gave special recognition and prizes to the person who could upsell the most. The customer would say, "Only a buck more for unlimited amounts of popcorn and soda?! I'm in!" And they often were. I know that I've given into this gimmick too. And while some people would come back for their refills, many didn't. Some left with only half-eaten buckets. So why did they upgrade?

Just in case. Just in case they wanted more. And the prestige of having an endless amount of popcorn. But if you're like me, I want my money's worth, and I'd probably try to eat two buckets just to make sense of my purchase. And my hips don't need half a bucket's worth of buttery smooth movie theater popcorn, let alone multiple buckets. So, there's that, too.

But that's what drives our upgrades, right?

What if I don't upgrade or buy the bigger, better thing, and then I miss out on something? Like, what if I run out of popcorn and really wish I had more? I won't risk it. Cue #FOMO.

Or what if that new iPhone has a new drone feature and I miss out on all of the awesome pictures I might ever want to take of an aerial view of my life? Gotta get it.

Yet we can have everything and still have nothing.

If whatever drives us to keep going for the newer things were ever satisfied, we could stop. But all of the mess of the actual stuff, what it costs financially, what it costs emotionally, and the endless pit of our soul that still cries out "not enough" is exhausting on all counts.

In *Walden*, Thoreau says, "The cost of a thing is not what the market will bear but what the individual must bear because of it: it is 'the amount of what I will call life which is required to be exchanged for it, immediately or in the long run.'"[2] He goes on to say that one of his greatest skills has been to want little.

Maybe the new car cost $25,000. Thoreau would ask how much life you lived, how much time you spent working, how much emotional energy was spent, building that $25,000 for the car. And not only the amount of life it took to get the car, but to keep it.

This is true for every item or service or opportunity we have the chance to involve in our lives. It's never as simple as the dollar amount.

And, as global statistics show, the harder we work and the more we consume, the less we seem to enjoy our lives. Nations with relatively little have shown higher levels of satisfaction than nations with a great abundance of wealth.

> In 1957, when economist John Galbraith was about to describe the United States as the Affluent Society, Americans' per person income, expressed in today's dollars, was $8,700. Today it is $20,000. Compared to 1957, we are now "the doubly affluent society"—with double what money buys. We have twice as many cars per person. We eat out two and a half times as often. Compared to the late 1950's when few Americans had dishwashers, clothes dryers, or air conditioning, most do today. So, believing that it's very important to be very well off, are

we now happier? Since 1957, the number of Americans who say they are "very happy" has declined from 35 to 32 percent. Meanwhile, the divorce rate has doubled, the teen suicide rate has nearly tripled, the violent crime rate has nearly quadrupled (even after the recent decline), and depression has mushroomed. These facts of life explode a bombshell underneath our society's materialism: Economic growth has provided no boost to human morale. When it comes to psychological well-being, it is not the economy, stupid."[3]

I've heard that the average person believes they will be happy with $1,000 more a month.[4] But when they get it, they find it's still not enough. *If only I had $1,000 more per month.* Even the wealthiest people deal with the "but if I had just a little more" mentality. They seem to have everything by external appearances, but it still feels lacking. How about the person who can hardly pay their bills? Wouldn't $1,000 more per month *actually* make *them* happy? Yeah, for a minute. They'll feel relief from the burden of late bills. But just like most people, they'll eventually get comfortable with what they have and begin spending more, finding their happiness is *just* out of reach…

What was supposed to bring us happiness and freedom from worry, brings frustration, stress, conflict, financial debt, etc. So many of us find ways to spend just a little more than what we have. This is evidenced by the plethora of stuff in our homes, in our storage units, on our computer drives. While we should have more than enough, we still have not-enough. And what we do have? Well, we can't even find it to appreciate it anymore.

"Over the course of our lifetime, we will spend a total of 3,680 hours or 153 days searching for misplaced items. The research found we lose up to nine items every day—or 198,743 in a lifetime. Phones, keys, sunglasses, and paperwork top the list…Many knew that untidiness and poor memory led to them losing track of items, with more than half wishing they were more organised. An unfortunate fourteen people said they spend over an hour every day looking for things they've misplaced."[5] And these are the things we need regularly. What about all of the things we've bought that stay tucked away in boxes, under the bed, lost under a pile? They no longer satisfy, partly because we have so much, we can't appreciate it anymore! Then, instead of giving us the joy they promised at the checkout counter, they're sucking the life out of us.

THE ABUNDANCE OF LESS

Treehugger founder Graham Hill is a great example of someone who went from "normal" to "extremely wealthy" and experienced having it all and finding that it wasn't everything he'd thought it was. Young in his life, he sold his startup company, Siteworks, for more than he thought he'd ever make in a lifetime. He immediately bought the big house, the car, the gadgets and gizmos, and filled the house. He said, "My success and the things it bought quickly changed from novel to normal. Soon I was numb to it all. The new Nokia phone didn't excite me or satisfy me. It didn't take long before I started to wonder why my theoretically upgraded life didn't feel any better and why I felt more anxious than before. My life was unnecessarily complicated. There were lawns to mow, gutters to clear, floors to vacuum, roommates to manage (it seemed nuts to have such a big, empty house), a car to insure, wash, refuel, repair, and register, and tech to set up and keep working…My house and my things were my new employers for a job I had never applied for."

Hill goes on to share about an experience that completely changed his view on stuff. He lived in Barcelona, renting a small flat, and having none of his luxuries along with him. He was free to travel all over with only his backpack. He felt more free, energized, and creative than he could in his overwhelmingly stressful home. He went on to say that his experience showed "that after a certain point, material objects have a tendency to crowd out the emotional needs they are meant to support."[6]

"Intuitively," said Hill, "we know that the best stuff in life isn't stuff at all, and that relationships, experiences and meaningful work are the staples of a happy life." He now lives in a 420-square-foot-home with his six shirts and his ten salad bowls. He doesn't own a single CD or DVD anymore. It took him "fifteen years, a great love, and a lot of travel to get rid of all the inessential things [he] had collected and live a bigger, better, richer life with less."

There's definitely a part of me that longs for such freedom. I spent my single years living just like he is. I had a mattress on the floor of a room I rented. I had a bag and most of my stuff could fit in it. I could pick up and move in less than an hour. I lived all over the place and *loved* it. When I married, my husband was twenty-nine and had lived as a bachelor for some time. He had a small household of things that I moved right into, with my one bag. (Well, and my parents dropped off a box or two of childhood toys and yearbooks they'd been storing in their garage. They needed the space.) Then, his parents offered to let us buy their house—a large house. A house with a mother-in-law suite attached. Like, a house with another small house attached. Four bedrooms, two living rooms, a den, a separate dining room, a dining nook, a kitchen, three bathrooms, a laundry room, and a large backyard in a culd-e-sac. Within two years I went from living happily in one room with a bag, to a two-bedroom apartment minimally furnished, to an ENTIRE HOUSE with a side mini-house. While we were in the process of moving into said house, and his parents were in the process of moving out, a sudden tragedy took his parents from the home. Not only did we have *the house*, but now we had our apartment worth of stuff, and their whole house worth of stuff.

So, let me sum that up for you again. One room and a bag, to an apartment with my husband's stuff (and my bag), to a house with our apartment amount of stuff, to a house with a house *and* an additional apartment's worth of stuff—and my bag.

Talk about stress. I mean, the tragedy alone was enough stress for one lifetime. (You can read our memoir of the tragedy in *While We Slept: Finding Hope and Healing After Homicide*.) But the sheer amount of *stuff* that we inherited was beyond my ability to cope with. And remember, this is the mother-in-law I already mentioned from the Depression Era. With her fifteen toothbrushes that were on sale. And the ten-plus jars of jelly she'd saved for eight years (her mother had made them and, after she'd passed away, my mother-in-law was unable to throw the jelly away. (See "sentimentality" in Chapter Four.)

Well, and because of the way in which we'd inherited this house full of things, the extended family members all wanted to approve *anything* we wanted to sell or give away before we actually did so. I get it, I really do. There were family heirlooms. Collections. Lots of stuff. And as an outsider to the family, I would likely throw something of great value away, not knowing its worth to the family. (Actually, I did this once—my husband left for a few days and I wanted to make him an art studio in the garage as a surprise. While he was gone, a bunch of our friends came over. We cleared out and sorted the garage, painted, bought fun little things, and made a great space. Oh, but to make that great space, I had to donate about eight pieces of luggage. I mean, we were only two people, we didn't need eight pieces of luggage. WELLLLLL it ends up that one or two of those luggage pieces were brought over by his grandfather when he immigrated from Denmark—whoops. The surprise ended up getting me in big trouble.)

Eleven years later, we've moved across the world (getting rid of ninety-five percent of our things) only to have a bunch again. Being a family of six doesn't help, and neither does the good-hearted (albeit sneaky) giving I mentioned in Chapter Two.

I miss living out of a bag.

And I can stay in a state of loss as I look around my house and realize how quickly what goes *out* can come back in, *or* I can do something about it. But how can I, one person, really make an ongoing, lasting change? I'll tell you how in the next chapter.

---

[1] 10 Hidden Secrets of Starbucks' Global Success, including insights into marketing and behavioral economics by Michael Chibba, August 21, 2015. https://www.linkedin.com/pulse/10-hidden-secrets-starbucks-global-success-including-insights-chibba accessed on 10/29/16

[2] Walden by Henry David Thoreau, August 9, 1854

[3] The Disconnect Between Wealth and Wellbeing: It's Not the Economy, Stupid, by David G Myers, https://www.edge.org/response-detail/11208 accessed 10/29/16

[4] Wiblin, R. (2018, December 10). Everything You Need to Know About Whether Money Makes You Happy. Retrieved June 20, 2020, from https://80000hours.org/articles/money-and-happiness/

[5] Lost Something Already Today? Misplaced Items Cost Us Ten Minutes a Day, March 21, 2012, http://www.dailymail.co.uk/news/article-2117987/Lost-today-Misplaced-items-cost-minutes-day.html accessed 10/29/16

[6] Living With Less. A Lot Less. by Graham Hill, March 9, 2013, http://www.nytimes.com/2013/03/10/opinion/sunday/living-with-less-a-lot-less.html accessed 10/29/16

Blog Post—June—Immersion Blender Freebie

This is such a fun story and I can't believe I haven't shared it yet! But since I used my "new" immersion blender tonight for our soup (and loved every minute of it), I saw it as only appropriate to write about this gift...while my soup simmers.

Awhile back, I had decided that I would like an immersion blender. I make a corn tortilla soup that requires blending, and more than a few times I have burned myself as splashes of boiling soup attack me as I pour it into my *regular* blender, which, by the way, doesn't fit the whole of my soup. Needless to say, watching friends blend their soups so beautifully and cleanly created some blender-envy. I decided to see what I could find used. This led to a lot of nothing as it seems that many people are not looking to get rid of their immersion blenders (who can blame them?).

So, one day I get on Freecycle and see a woman offering kitchen things. I check it out and sure enough, at the bottom of her list, is an immersion blender. FREE! I promptly send her an email requesting it. After I sent my email, I looked at the time—she had posted the day before. I thought to myself, *There is* no *way that is still available a day later.* Then I realized that my messages were flipped! They were showing older to newer! Sure enough, once I corrected my posts...there it was, the fatal "Taken: Kitchen stuff." I sadly emailed the person back saying how sorry I was that I'd missed the "Taken" post and to disregard my message. Thinking it was over, I moved on with my life.

However, I received a reply email stating that while all of the kitchen stuff *was* gone...the immersion blender was still available and sitting on her porch waiting for me (address included and all!) You can bet that I jumped in my car and drove right over to pick up my beloved gift from God.

It's crazy how often we think that God doesn't care about these small things in our life. And really, in relation to all the tragedies in the world, He shouldn't. But what a blessing to know that in His omnipresence and omnipotence, He can care about the silliest things that my heart ponders. And then to take the time to respond! Had my Freecycle posts been in order, I *never* would have emailed that woman about her kitchen stuff! So many providential things in place with an eventual leading to my "new" immersion blender. And tonight, as in so many nights yet to come, I am extremely grateful for His thoughtfulness, and the thoughtfulness of the woman giving it away!

So, to all of you who wonder if God cares about the *big* things in your life, let alone the small things, know that He does. And though not every answer is a "yes" or even comes in the way we expect, He does love to give His kids good gifts. May you continue to be inspired to allow God to meet your needs!

Chapter 6

How Can I Change the World? Or Even Empty that Drawer?

So how do we make a difference in all of this?

How do we reduce our "carbon footprint?"

How do I, one single person, make any difference in the world at all?

Also, how can anyone who truly loves me expect me to go into my daughter's room? It's a disaster in there! Just looking at it makes me turn right around and seek out some brain-numbing activity that can erase the horror of how she lives. I can't even begin to muster the energy that her room requires—again. Because I've given it *hours upon hours* of my life, and it takes her no time at all to return it to its can't-see-the-floor-or-the-bed-or-your-brother kind of way. Okay, it's mostly books and clothes, but still. You'd be amazed at what an awful carpet all of that makes.

If I can't even muster up the energy to make a difference in *her* room, how can I ever make a difference in the ozone or the melting ice glaciers?

For starters, I need to talk myself down off that cliff. Some people are motivated by dreaming that big, and cheers to them. I, however, need baby steps. How does one eat an elephant? One bite at a time.

So, we start with something small. Something we can manage. Maybe it's one drawer in the house. Maybe it's a choice to *not* buy something you would have normally purchased. Maybe it's to send money to a charity instead of on another belt (thinking of you, Priscilla Shirer!*).[1] We *can* choose to change how we contribute to the nation of excess and the culture of convenience, even if it's just one thing.

I had to do the same thing with a lifestyle change we made with food. When I read *The Maker's Diet* by Jordan Rubin, I wept. It was so much information and I finished it realizing how much I'd been lied to about food in my life! No wonder I'd always been chunky! (It had nothing to do with the Pepsi or chicken nuggets though, right, Jordan?)[2] Once I could focus again, I realized that I was too overwhelmed to do a complete overhaul of the way we ate. *But* I could change one thing. I could trade out my vegetable oil for coconut oil.

That switch ended up pretty easy. So, I decided to try another switch: eggs. I'd buy happy-chicken eggs. And it ends up that happy chickens lay big, delicious, vibrant-yolked eggs. I moved on to milk. Then seasonings. And before I knew it, we were eating the foods we understood to be healthiest for our bodies. We even ended up doing a few of his hardcore food detoxes.

One of the things that kept inspiring me to make changes was the impact each change made on our health. We could feel the difference in our energy levels. We watched pounds shed away. We had clearer minds. And our food was actually more delicious. Each positive change in our lives spurred us to try one more new thing.

I won't lie and say we've always done it perfectly. I still love me some French fries and schnitzel! But nine or so years later, much of how we choose to eat is still based on that plan. And because we've informed ourselves, when I make a food decision contrary to what's best for me, I know exactly what I'm bringing on—tiredness, decreased immunity, muddled thinking, on and on.

Changing our consumer lifestyle is not much different. The more changes you make, the more you'll experience new freedom. The first steps are always painful. Getting rid of things is like cutting off appendages sometimes. Or like losing a pet. You have an emotional attachment to some of the items you need to let go of. So just choose one and do it well. Shoot, give it a ceremony, I don't care. But do it.

In our case, we decided we could try a whole year of not buying anything new. When I see it written there, it doesn't seem like a big deal. "Oh right, just go to the thrift store and buy your stuff. Or don't buy stuff at all. I could do that, easy-peasy." And maybe *you* could. But I had four children, sometimes more, as a foster parent. A British research found that the average 10-year-old owns 238 toys but plays with just twelve daily.[3] Another study showed that 3.1% of the world's children live in America, but they own 40 percent of the toys consumed globally.[4] That same study noted that women who are bothered by clutter show increased levels of the stress hormone Cortisol, while their male counterparts were unaffected. Ladies, we are not crazy, they really are unaffected.

So, four children times an average of 238 toys per child—and that's just kids. Choosing to tackle a buy-nothing-new year was sounding pretty good to me, since I hate having so much stuff. But then the sewing machine broke down in the first few days of our challenge. And my husband's Bible flew off the car. And we lost the key to our fireplace (which did something important). And then I was given a gift card to Target. It was like a big fat test in meeting our "needs" in a brand-new way, and it couldn't involve our usual late-night run to Target or a quick hop onto Amazon.

This was how we were choosing to make a difference, even if it only mattered to our family. Shoot, even if it only mattered to me. And already, it was under fire.

I'm not asking you to take the challenge (though it would be *awesome* if you did—can you imagine how we really *could* change the country if we all stopped buying new things for an entire year? I think the world would stop. And the U.S. would have to get really creative about how to keep the economy booming. Or, maybe the country would save a bunch of money too since it wouldn't need to produce nearly as much stuff, and we could pay off all of our debts. Hmmm). But I'm not asking you to do that.

But I *am* asking you to do *something*. Use up your freezer items and get rid of that giant freezer that's sucking up electricity to store your excessive food. (Or at least unplug it and save the electricity until you *really* need the freezer space, like for when you're having a birthday ice cream buffet and you need twenty-nine tubs of ice cream). Go one week without buying anything new. Sew the hole in your shirt instead of buying a new one. Buy from a local artist. Hand-make your next gift or card. Find someone who could really use the extra (fill in the blank) that you have. Refugees moving into town? They need all sorts of stuff! Give them some of yours (but not your junk. Remember my Lesvos experience in Chapter Three? Yeah, don't do that to people).

There are so many ways that we can take one step toward being people who are free, who are happy, who live with less stress, who share the wealth instead of hoard it, and who aren't slaves to our possessions. So many ways you can take one tiny bite into that huge elephant and begin experiencing gratitude for the things you have and contentment bigger than your walk-in closet. Which one will you try today?

HOW CAN I CHANGE THE WORLD? OR EVEN EMPTY THAT DRAWER?

1. Sometimes you add someone's name in a book as if you know them and somehow they're going to read your book. I mean, I read hers, after all. Then again, she is a public speaker, author, actress, and she has a gazillion fans. Still, in a recent Bible Study of hers that I completed, she talked about having too much stuff. One of her weaknesses are belts. Maybe it's yours too and I can give you a shout-out next time.
2. There I go again. Name dropping like we're old buds and he's going to be reading my book. I mean, I've read about three of his books, so I feel like we're old friends. I wonder if there's a DSM-5 diagnosis for people who drop famous names like they're buds?
3. University of California TV Series Looks at Clutter Epidemic in Middle-Class American Homes, http://www.uctv.tv/RelatedContent.aspx?RelatedID=301, accessed 10/29/16
4. Ten Year Olds Have £7000 Worth of Toys but Play with Just £330, October 20, 2010, http://www.telegraph.co.uk/finance/newsbysector/retailandconsumer/8074156/Ten-year-olds-have-7000-worth-of-toys-but-play-with-just-330.html, accessed 10/29/16

Blog Post—April—Birthday

It's true. My daughter is turning one. Fortunately, it seems I've picked a theme that a lot of people can help with! We are having a Luau barbecue to celebrate her year of life. I have had so many people lend and give us leis, grass skirts, tablecloths, lanterns—it's been amazing. I've even found leis at a thrift store! It is slowly coming together and I'm so excited to see what the end result will be. I even found a grass skirt *for* my one-year-old! Oh, watch out for those pictures! Goodness.

Anyway, here we are in month four and still sticking to our resolution really well. It's amazing to see how little we need. In fact, we recently purged our house and had a yard sale. We made just over $100 on things we really would have *paid* people to take away! The yard sale went something like this:

Customer: "How much for this (fill in the blank)?"

Us: "Five dollars"

Customer: "Oh," and starts to walk away and look around.

Us: "But how much will you take it for?"

Customer: "One dollar."

Us: "Excellent! It's yours!"

We couldn't be talked down too low. The rest was donated to a local thrift store that I found on accident. The employer was out of tax-deductible receipts and I didn't care—I just wanted to get rid of the leftover stuff. That's the thrift store where I found two leis. He let me have them for free.

All that said, it seems our hearts are changing with this resolution in some interesting ways. Not only do we not want *more* but we are finding we don't even really want or need all that we *have*. We are living on our own excess in so many ways. It's been so freeing to clear a bunch out. I feel round two coming on! Here's what we got rid of (in general): three dressers, two end tables, diaper changing table, baby video monitor, a bike, two bookshelves, a bar stool, lots of clothes, broken skateboard (gave that away to someone who wanted to buy it!), and lots of kitchen stuff. One woman even asked if we had any towels for sale. So, we pulled out *all* of our rags and let her pick what she wanted! It was fun to run in our house and try to find things that people were looking for. A lot of it was just given away too. It's amazing we made any money at all. One family was looking for baby dishes, so I ran in and pulled out my pantry for her to look through.

I pray that if there is anything hindering your freedom in this life, that you would be reminded that this is a hotel on our way to our permanent home. Your life is so short in the light of eternity. LET IT GO! This continues to be a lesson to myself—honestly, even as I look at my cluttered desk top right now. MOVE IT ON!

Blessings to you each as you endeavor to free up your lives however God leads you and to live on the plenty that we have!

Chapter 7

How to Start

Starting can feel daunting. Overwhelming. In fact, I think if, in 2010, I'd really stopped to think about what I was stepping into, I would have over-analyzed it and frozen with indecision. But the reality was, I was on a mission and no one around me was doing anything like it. I was a pioneer.

So, I started with what I *could* do. I decided to see if anyone else was feeling the same way I was. Were there other people wishing they could live more in community, less reliant on mass-produced, over-produced, commercial *stuff*?

I hoped so.

In fact, at the time, a quick yellow-pages search (I know) revealed around twenty second-hand stores in my city. I saw numerous signs every weekend pointing to yard sales and flea markets. Clearly others were aware that stuff needed to *go*.

Yet, as quickly as that stuff was out the door, another load of stuff from the nearest sale or the you-must-have-this-to-survive commercial was unpacking into the corners of the house. How could I begin to make a dent in this crazy situation? Well…

Do what *you* can do.

Find like-minded people. Find the people who are tired of living with so much stuff, so much clutter, so much *noise* and join forces. They might be in your social circle, your neighborhood, your church, your social media community. Join together and start with yourselves!

That's what I did.

Initially I joined Craigslist and Yahoo Groups. For those of you younger than Facebook, Yahoo Groups and Craigslist were online portals where you could post ads and meet people. In fact, Craigslist was started by, you got it, Craig! In 1995, Craig began using his email list to keep friends and family informed about local events. He was new to the Bay Area of California and had seen how the Internet could be used in a friendly, social, community-oriented way. Word of mouth led people to ask to join his email list. A year later, it was a Web-based site. Today it's in over seventy countries.

One lonely dude decided to reach out and *bring belonging* to the people around him. I imagine he figured he wasn't alone in feeling new and isolated and left-out-of-the-loop, so he'd share what he was learning with others. And it took off.

Start where you are. Find like-minded people.

Another place I connected with like-minded people was Yahoo Groups. For many years, Yahoo hosted online discussion groups, chat rooms, forums, and the like. Only in 2020 did Yahoo close access to all of the discussion groups. But before that, I found some Buy-and-Sell groups. They ran similar to what we might have on Facebook…members could post in the forum and leave comments. Moderators often went through and deleted posts or sent rants in emails about all of the rule-breakers.

However, I found both of these sites to be insufficient. Craigslist, at least in my area, had quickly become known as dangerous and unreliable. A number of people had arrived to specified locations to pick up items, only to go missing, *dead*, or have creepy experiences. There just wasn't a lot of monitoring *who* was posting and if they were real people or mass murderers. (A quick Google search pulls up a number of these incidents.) I didn't have any horrible experiences with Craigslist personally, but in my circles, most people didn't go alone. I certainly wasn't trying to *die* to find or give used things.

Thus, I leaned more into Yahoo Groups, but even this was unreliable and, at times, felt threatening. I might find an item and show up—only to find it dirty or broken. And many times, in the Buy-and-Sell groups I followed, moderators would get frustrated with people breaking the rules and send emails full of ranting and railing against the evildoers. It left me feeling unsure of whether I was the only trustworthy person trying to buy and sell used.

This left me to my own devices. I wanted to share this experience with people I trusted, in a community with which I was comfortable, among friends and family with whom I might also benefit.

Facebook was relatively new, at least to the general population, at the time of our experiment in 2010. Yet I'd seen enough to know that it was bringing people together in a unique way. It wasn't like the faceless, public sites like Craigslist and Yahoo Groups. It gave me control over my friendship circles, connected me with people I'd thought long lost, and brought the possibility of sharing photos and statuses with this chosen group of people. There were also groups, where you could invite people to join you around a shared theme. Who knew, back then, how Facebook would grow to *change the world* and how we interact, get our news, share our opinions, and promote our brands. All I knew back then was I wanted a safe place to offer my give-away goods and find what we might need during this year.

So, I created one of the first (*the* first?) Facebook sales/swap groups. I named the group "Living Hebrews 13:5" based on a verse that held great meaning for me. "Keep your lives free from the love of money and be content with what you have, because God has said, 'Never will I leave you; never will I forsake you.'" I know there are a handful of other verses that would have supported this vision, but I loved the foundation of this one: remaining free from loving money (greed) and finding contentment in what I have (trust) *because* God would never leave me. If I could grasp the depth of that kind of security, I could release my false sense of control around having *stuff* and what it could do for me.

Being raised on welfare, in a sometimes-single parent home, fully aware that the next meal wasn't always guaranteed, formed how I lived as an adult. Not on the surface level, but deep beneath. I could both live on very little (because then I had less to lose) or on *a lot* (because then I was "secure.") When I lived with a lot, it gave me a sense of pride—I could give to *my* kids what I didn't necessarily have growing up. Not just the stuff itself, but the assurance of every meal, every need, all the time. It gave me a sense of power to provide.

Now, being able to provide is *huge* and definitely, we should provide for our families! But the internal conversations in *me* around the purpose of stuff were unhealthy and ultimately fed a deep fear that someday I'd go without. Then what? The reality is, in my case, though the next meal wasn't always assured…*I never missed a meal.* It always showed up. I know that's not every kid's story. But it's mine. And I'm impacted by it. So, choosing to lean into the provision of God over my fear of powerlessness was a win, and a reminder I need often.

So, my Facebook group, *Living Hebrews 13:5*, was started. I invited a bunch of my friends and went to bed. I had no idea what would become of it. If anyone else felt the need for it. But I hoped.

And I slept.

The next morning, I woke up to nearly one hundred members. By the end of the day it was up to a couple hundred. By the end of the week, we were pushing one thousand members from my local community; *and they were using it!* See, here's the thing. I could have set up an incredible idea, but unless the people *used* it, it would have been just another empty group.

But clearly, at least one thousand other people loved the idea and were immediately offering and searching. It was beautiful. I was *blown away.* And, unique to some other Buy-and-Sell groups today, I purposefully decide to keep the group around one thousand people. I didn't want to lose the familiarity we had with one another (there's one to two degrees of separation among members) and the sense that this was local community supporting local community.

News of my new group flew through the grapevine. Soon I had Facebook friends around the country asking me how I'd done it so they could set one up in *their* community. It was amazing! Groups like mine spread like wildfire. People began joining with each other in upcycling—re-using or repurposing things instead of going out to buy the next new promise-of-happiness gadget.

Now, this might not seem unusual to you. Facebook's Marketplace has been around since 2016. (Ironically, Facebook launched a Marketplace feature in 2007 but it totally flopped). In 2015, Facebook added the ability, within a post, to choose "For Sale" and list it as an item for purchase. I remember when this was added to my Living Hebrews group, thinking, *Brilliant! They see the value of using Facebook for groups like mine!* Of course, it took a full five years after the start of my group, but *still*, it was movement to support social selling within the safety of one's community. When Facebook launched Marketplace for a second time in 2016, already *450 million* were visiting Facebook Buy-and-Sell groups like mine.[1] It was about time they launched Marketplace, which now allows people outside of a particular group to search an item within a particular radius of their choosing.

But thinking back to 2010, when Facebook had been cycling people into the once college-based platform through beta-testing, and the idea was new and growing, you can imagine what it meant to have a tool that could bring people together so uniquely for nearly the first time. And, to already have one thousand people in my community who wanted to use it for collaboration and connection—amazing.

I did a poll in Living Hebrews, in addition to groups I later joined, on the impact of having a Facebook group such as these. The comments were inspiring and heart-warming:

I asked the group, "Why did you join this group?"

> "To be part of a more trusted selling community. I love that within this group there is only one to two degrees of separation."

> "To sell things I didn't need any longer and to find things I *did* need without having to go to a yard sale."

> "A friend invited me and I liked the idea of sharing and selling to/buying from 'friends of a friend' (which seems much safer and more reliable than Craigslist)."

I then asked group members what they loved most about the group:

> "Seeing smiles on people's faces when they buy something of mine at a great price!"

> "I love that I can TRUST this group and people keep their word. I give people my address and meet at my house. I know that no one will scam me here."

> "I feel more connected to the community. Meeting people that I normally would have no reason to interact with."

> "I've actually gotten to know people that I never would have met otherwise."

> "Well, I think to some extent it restored my faith in people. I'm probably a skeptical person, but this group has a decent amount of really nice folks."

"Cleaning out and minimizing = a more organized and happy me; cash for my kids when they sell stuff = they're willing to get rid of old stuff, too."

"It's been encouraging to see that "junk" has ended up being a treasure to the refugee community that came flooding in starting in 2015."

"Last year we were in a pretty tight financial spot and I needed clothes but couldn't afford them. Someone offered free stuff at just the right time and blessed me hugely!"

"Finding our home was the greatest benefit! Rented it sight unseen, except for a few pics."

"We bought a bed from someone I had never met, but we had a lot of mutual friends in the Christian community in Fresno. It was a great experience and she even let us use her truck to take the bed."

"I once posted on the kiddie version on the FB group that I was in need of maternity clothes and would be willing to buy work-appropriate pants. It was the last six weeks of my second (and last) pregnancy and my old pregnancy clothes were not fitting like they used to. Not wanting to spend a lot of money for only 6 weeks of wearing, I gave the FB group a shot. Someone actually gave me several pairs of maternity pants for free. I was grateful and they were glad to off load the stuff."

"I love meeting someone face-to-face that I've only known on the Buy-and-Sell group. Also, I have a first edition Nook. The original cover was getting old and shredding, but it was hard enough finding any covers for the old model, let alone to let go of the cover I loved in one of my favorite colors. But the cover was in terrible shape, so

I threw it out. The next week someone posted the exact same cover—brand new—for free! That was awesome!"

Like anything, groups like these have their incredible benefits, but also bumps and bruises along the way. I asked the members of a few groups, "What are some downsides you've experienced in a group like this?" They said:

"Too many people joined and the idea of Free-cycling became null. People started overpricing their items hoping to make some money instead of have a yard sale. Now it seems that it is just another Buy-Sell-Trade site."

"When people don't follow the rules."

"When they sell trashy stuff."

"I find it frustrating that people can be a little more rude in their interactions online than (I hope) they'd be in face-to-face interactions, because this group is still the best way to stay informed in the community."

I think both the positive and negative aspects of the Facebook Buy-and-Sell groups all point to one major need: community. People praised the way community supported them in times of need. And begrudged when the community got too big, too greedy, or too careless in interactions. People want a safe place to share and be shared with.

Flash forward to 2012. We had (*spoiler alert!*) survived our 2010 year of buying only used things and gotten rid of at least 90% of our belongings. We packed our family of six and the last of what we owned and moved to Germany. We moved to volunteer at a school called Black Forest Academy which exists to provide high-quality education to families providing humanitarian aid work around the world. We help families in Africa, the Middle East, Asia, and Europe who are digging wells to provide clean water, running orphanages, offering community development, traveling medical aides, on and on. It's a privilege…and it cost us everything comfortable about our lives.

That aside, when we arrived, we found a whole community of people who'd planted themselves around the school. Many of them were staff, like my husband. And many were organizations overseeing the work of their members around the world. They'd established regional offices in this little German village in order to send their own children to BFA while supporting their members in more isolated locations. This is important to know, because the source of information was a *corkboard* in the hallway of the main offices of the school. Where only a fraction of the people regularly walked.

After having run Living Hebrews for a couple of years, I was a bit astounded to see how rudimentary the community-communication system was for such a high-quality establishment. Little want ads littered the board. Photos of a bed for sale, a house for rent, shoes to give cluttered the wall. I stared in disbelief. And I simultaneously did *not* want to be the "new staff member" trying to make major overhauls to a system that had been in a place a *long time.*

Too long.

So, I rallied new friends of mine who'd been in the community much longer than I had. They loved the idea. Together, with their support, I started the Kandern Area Flohmärkte.

It took off.

It took off like I'd offered ice water to parched desert travelers.

It suddenly made space for *belonging.* There had been an inadvertent divide between those who worked on the school campus and those who didn't (thus, having limited to no access to the cork board). Now *everyone* could participate equally. It made us feel like *one* complete body of expatriates, versus random groupings of people assigned to our various offices and positions.

It brought *support.* People came and left this community regularly. The highly transient nature and the poor access to communication and support left people re-creating the "wheel" regularly. Now, old-timers or less-new-timers could share tips, ideas, and offer practical guidance to newbies. In fact, the school's HR reached out to me about adding incoming staff before their arrival, so they could get questions answered as they packed up their homes around the world in preparation for coming to our community. "Should I bring my muffin tin?" "Can I get Nyquil there?" "Will my fitted bed sheet fit the German mattress?" We were able to help save incomers tons of money, time, and unnecessary stress because of the Facebook community. And not just because of the exchange of *goods* but because of the emotional, physical, mental, and even spiritual support that the Facebook group offered.

This particular Facebook group in Germany now hosts about 600 people from the surrounding area and has broken into two branches of itself: The Buy-and-Sell aspect (which gets very busy each summer as people transition in or out) and the community-help aspect where we answer questions like, "Will the grocery stores be open this Monday during the holiday?" Or, "Why are there people dressed in animal skins and bells walking through town?"

And I'm happy to report that the cork board has come down. In its place the walls are now adorned with the artwork of our very gifted students.

So what does this mean for *you*?

How do you get started?

Well, for one, you can search Facebook for an already-going group in your area. By now, groups like these are as common as air. You can also utilize the Marketplace for finding things you need within a range of your home.

And Facebook isn't the only option. While not holding the same community feel, you can easily buy and sell used goods on sites like Amazon, eBay, Boohoo, and Craigslist. I also discovered the Next Door App while living in California one year. This provided an opportunity for neighbors in the same vicinity to swap/sell/buy, share about neighborhood information, alert others to any suspicious activity, report a missing (or found) pet, on and on. It was pretty cool!

But maybe you want to start something within your own community. Here are some easy steps to get you going.

1. **Create a group on Facebook.** The way to do this changes from time to time so you can Google it or simply click on "Groups" and look for instructions.

2. **Set great expectations.** This might include things like: leave it on the porch, leave it clean, be responsive, delete your post once its resolved, be generous, avoid frequent self-promotion, etc.

3. **Find someone to help you moderate.** While I haven't found this to be terribly time-consuming, it's really nice to have a partner or small team to help you with unexpected situations that might come up. Plus, then there's not one "bad guy" if you have to enforce a group guideline or remove someone from the community. It's an admin-team decision.

4. **Send invites to your local friends/community**. Odds are, you know plenty of people in your area who would totally jam on this with you. You can control who and how many. Keep it as intimate as you want or grow it to include anyone in your city. But it starts with who you know and making space for them to start engaging.

5. **Be the first one to give!** It's always easy to be the first one to ask for something. But be the first to give instead. Model for the community, from the start, a spirit of giving and generosity. In this spirit, everyone ends up with what they need, plus hearts full and inspired by humanity.

While starting can feel overwhelming, the end result is worth every minute of discomfort. I'm so glad, back in 2010, when I felt pretty alone and unsure of myself in this new project, that I didn't let me insecurities (trust me, I've got plenty) or fear of discomfort (yep, I have a healthy dose of that too) get in the way of what has become life-impacting for so many. You might feel tempted to let someone else get it going. Or maybe they already have! You get to just show up and bring all the good that you have to offer, maybe even being the answer to someone else's desperate prayer of need. The opportunities are endless. Pick yours and get going!

In the next few chapters, I'll share *how it went*. The lessons learned, the challenges we faced, our failures (uh-huh, totally failed a few times) and how my life has never been the same since.

---

[1] Constine, J. (2016, October 03). Facebook launches Marketplace, a friendlier Craigslist. Retrieved May 17, 2020, from https://techcrunch.com/2016/10/03/facebook-marketplace-2/

Blog Post—January—The Blessing of Sharing

There are a number of thrift stores in our city. I looked in the online yellow pages and there were about twenty listed. There were some I noticed that *weren't* listed. Here is my opinion. Salvation Army has a really great ministry and service to the community, one that you see the fruit of. I've even had dear friends participate in their programs. Their prices are good, and they offer sales all the time. Goodwill, I have found, is too highly priced and not as service oriented—at least, not in such visible ways as Salvation Army. Go where you want, but I have found a number of things at Goodwill that were *more* expensive than the *same* item next door at Walmart. When I brought that to the attention of the staff (on both occasions) they told me to go shop at Walmart.

There are also great websites life half.com, ebay.com, amazon.com where you can get used items at a decent deal. Google will compare prices for you. Lots of great options!

Your best options, I believe, are your friends and family and local community. The blessing of sharing as a greater body is awesome! Just a taste of what the Church recorded in Acts must have experienced.

Now, on a slightly humorous note, I came home last night and found that I'd won a $25 gift card to Target. Of course I did! Instead of getting to use it on something new, like I would normally do, I will be buying toilet paper and diapers! Thank you, Lord, for your blessings which come in such timely ways!

Blog Post—February—Simplify

Today I had an appointment with our amazing chiropractor, Dr. Matt. During our family visit, he mentioned how they are trying to live more simply—buying less things.

He had no idea about our resolution.

We survived Valentine's day with hand-made valentine cards, homemade cookies, and leftover valentines from previous years (unused). The kids didn't lack anything in the way of traditions And Jeremy and I were forced to be a little creative, but in a way no less rich than previous years. Our real challenge will be with our oldest son's birthday party in a month. Hopefully we can pull the whole thing together under this resolution. I think we can!

Dr. Matt noted how much they were able to get used with the recent birth of their new daughter. They've had two sons, so they had nothing feminine on hand. But so many people have had things to give that they have had very little *need*.

I LOVE COMMUNITY!

Chapter 8

Immediate Gratification

One of the challenges we faced in this experiment was *waiting*. It felt like drudgery. I hadn't realized the extent to which I simply go and buy what I need or want when I want or need it. Or how often I stood in line and simply bought something on impulse. Target anyone? I always leave with too many $1 items I didn't even *know* I needed until I saw it *and* the amazing price.

It wasn't until I was in line for groceries and reached for a magazine. Or until we couldn't find the key to our fireplace (I know, it's a special fireplace) and *needed* a new one to get the ambience and heat we loved.

Waiting was hard.

Waiting felt like dying.

And it surprised me. I thought, as a mom to four-plus kids, that I'd become accustomed to waiting. I mean, I had to *wait* until nap times to get most things done. I had to *wait* to eat until everyone was fed and ready to go. I had to *wait* to pee until everyone was entertained enough and I could escape for a second. *Surely* I could wait for a new fireplace key to show up in one of these many Buy-and-Sell groups I was perusing.

But I didn't want to. I wanted it *now*. I wanted to do a quick search on Amazon and click "buy now." Don't put it in my cart and make me verify my purchase. Just send it Prime so I can have it tomorrow.

Why is waiting *so* hard?

Well, we are conditioned to avoid pain. Maybe we're also even designed to avoid pain. I'm sure it's a survival technique that has kept humanity on the planet. But needing my fireplace key and staying alive are different, aren't they?

This is where design and conditioning begin to blend and confuse. You see, we live in a culture of fast-paced, meet-our-need pressure. We are constantly inundated with how happy we'll be if we just have this or that. Simultaneously, we are fed how much *pain* we'll be in if we *don't* have this or that. We're sold Band-aid solutions all the time. What looks like a promise of pleasure and comfort really only provides a false sense of control and safety. Having that sports car is *not* going to make you look like the ripped stud driving it. Or the hot girl stroking it. It will, though, drain your paycheck to buy it, insure it, maintain it, and fuel it. But that's not what *they* tell us. Those anonymous *theys* who know just what we need to be as happy as happy can be.

We spend a *lot* of money to avoid discomfort. And all the while, what we don't realize, is that we are slowly killing our ability to find pleasure in the small, let alone the large, things. According to Dr. Archibald Hart, clinical psychologist and expert in behavioral psychology, our over-dedication to experiencing pleasure and avoiding pain is *actually* killing the pleasure center of the brain. In his book, *Thrilled to Death: How the Endless Pursuit of Pleasure Is Leaving Us Numb,* Dr. Hart unravels the science of our brain as it relates to a loss of experiencing pleasure and happiness, known as *anhedonia,* once a disorder only associated with serious emotional disorders but now seen regularly. In fact, it's a major cause of depression and anxiety disorders today.

Basically, the more we pursue pleasure, the more our brain requires to *experience* pleasure. Like a drug fix…the more you use a drug, the more you need to get the same high. In essence, we are thrilling our brains to death, robbing ourselves of the simple and beautiful joy of a sunrise, the view of the ocean, the smile of a friend. These things no longer provide the pleasure they once did, because we keep reaching for stronger and quicker access to pleasure, like scrolling through our social media feed, a "buy now" click while online shopping, Netflix movies at the press of a button, the thrills of gaming, social "engaging," and streams of entertainment at your fingertips through TikTok, Snapchat, Instagram, and Twitter.

We ruin our pleasure centers, making it harder to find pleasure in simple things. Are you surprised to find yourself totally oblivious to the sounds of nature around you? To the deep blues, purples, and oranges of a setting sun? Unmoved by the sound of water rushing through ravines or along a shore? If these still bring your soul a stillness and deep joy, then *yay!* Your pleasure center is still active—now keep it that way! If you've noticed that you're struggling to find pleasure in life, even from the things that used to provide it, consider how the downsides of instant gratification may have impacted you.

Essentially, living for our own gratification, as quickly satisfied as possible, returns us to the state of *babies*. Think about it! They are born, and for the first *long time,* everything they do, every sound they make, every waking moment is about *give me that now.* They cry until they get what they want. They cry to avoid pain and discomfort. Once they get it, they're appeased. Until they're not. And the cycle of cry-give-me, cry-give me starts again.

Avoiding pain means all of our energy and effort is devoted to *avoiding.* That means we have nothing left for chasing down dreams. For achieving our goals. For experiencing success. How many babies do you see accomplishing anything more than filling their tummies and getting clean diapers to replace dirty ones? That's the limit of their desires because life is spent avoiding pain.

Avoiding pain leads to the opposite of what makes our dreams come true.

Every unnecessary, pain-avoidant *no* gets in the way of our best yeses. Every time, to avoid pain, I refuse to step bravely into courage, into the space of fear and discomfort, and opt for easy…I lose something. Now, maybe you're thinking, *When I want something, and I want it now, it's a YES, not a NO!* Every fast yes is actually a *no* to something better and good. Every *fast* yes takes space from a better yes.

Early in our marriage, we were invited to a meal to accept a gift of Disneyland tickets we'd "won" or something to that effect. What we didn't know, was that this was a timeshare-type presentation meant to high-pressure sell us into their program. We felt uneasy by the bait-and-switch, in addition to the intensity of the one-on-two sales conversations they put us in at the conclusion of our meal. We were able to step aside and call a friend. Apparently, it was the wrong friend. We bought into the timeshare for the marked-down just-for-us price of $11,000, direct from the savings of newlyweds. Of course, once everything was signed, sealed, and transferred, we learned about the fine, fine print. For example, the yearly fee of $300 we'd have to pay to remain members of the "club." *Well shoot*, we thought, *we could have put aside $300 a year and saved up for a trip!* It was the largest "dumb tax" we've ever paid. It was years before we used the timeshare system because of how complicated accessing it was. We were tired of paying yearly fees on a program we couldn't figure out. When we looked into selling it, we were dismayed. People were trying to sell their timeshares all over the place, for as low as $1, in order to stop paying the yearly fees. Customers were begging potential buyers to take the burden off their hands. And now that was us.

My first thought was, *We could have bought this for ONE DOLLAR?!* And my second thought was, *We're stuck! We're going to have to* pay *someone to take this from us!* We decided we couldn't bear the humiliation of an $11,000 purchase we didn't use, so we hunkered down and figured it out, getting ourselves and our now-small family to Cabo San Lucas. It was great. It was a $12,000 trip, plus flights.

While we were vacationing there, a neighboring resort stopped us on the street and offered us lunch, $200, and a few other gifts to visit their resort. This time we knew *exactly* what we were getting into. We accepted. We were given a tour, a simple meal, and *three hours* of trying to convince us to buy into their timeshare-type program. We held to our no. It felt so good. They gave us the cash, a bottle of champagne, and a bizarre side door exit to a waiting car, which drove us fast and backwards down a long alley, where we were discarded on the side of the road. But we had done it! The $200 covered the tourist costs of our trip to Cabo, which we toasted with our glasses of champagne. We came home and sold our program for $1 to a guy collecting timeshares.

That hasty yes, the purchase of that timeshare program, robbed us of better yeses. I don't even know what they are because we missed them. But there were at least $12,000 worth of better yeses we passed by. It was a major Fail-Forward moment. That $12,000 lesson taught us the value of waiting, of saying no, of doing good research, and asking if this is our *best* yes.

Our hasty yes was really to avoid the pain of missing out on this "once-in-a-lifetime-opportunity." We were avoiding the pain of being a family who loves to travel and has to do it the "normal" way. We became slaves to our avoidance of discomfort and pain.

We *think* we are making the choice to buy that new outfit because it's on such a great sale, and won't we look so cute and save money at the same time? When in reality, your puppeteer of pain-avoidance has already conditioned you to *need* to look cute for affirmation, value, and acceptance. You slap down your credit card, not realizing your master has won once again, in control of your budget, your impulses, your every decision. You don't get to decide for yourself. Your pain-avoidance wins every time.

Just look at the typical American. Seventy-six percent of Americans live paycheck to paycheck[1]. Why is that? I'm sure there are a variety of reasons, but one major reason is that we spend more than we make. In 2018, Americans held nearly $14 trillion in combined household debt.[2] About 40% of the debt for people under the age of thirty-five is discretionary: entertainment, clothing, and other non-essential spending. Credit card debt alone, in the US, is around $1 trillion.[3] *insert shocked emoji face here* Okay, that's a lot of money, but what does that mean for the individual family? The statistics show that the average American family, in 2019, held $8,398 in credit card debt, averaging at least four cards per user. This doesn't even take into account student loans, mortgages, or car loans. This demonstrates our inability to say *no* to the monster. If we can't say "no" to our spending, and live within our means, then we aren't actually in control.

Am I making you uncomfortable? Don't worry, a cookie will make it better.

Speaking of cookies, did you know that 42% of Americans are obese?[4] While many programs have worked hard to reduce the number of overweight folks in America, the number continues to grow. Obesity has contributed to many of the leading causes of death in America, all health-related and many preventable, like heart disease, some cancers, diabetes, organ failure, etc. Why are we over-eating? Well, I'm sure there are many reasons but here are a few of my guesses:

1. We don't want to be hungry. We're afraid of discomfort and scarcity, so eat to avoid the pain and discomfort of hunger. Shauna Niequist, in her book *Bread and Wine: A Love Letter to Life Around the Table with Recipes* said, "I've always wanted to be thinner, and I've always loved to eat, and I felt betrayed by my appetite…My appetite is strong, powerful, precise, but for years and years I tried to pretend I couldn't hear it screaming in my ears. It wasn't lady-like, it wasn't proper. So, I pretended I wasn't hungry, pretended I'd already eaten, murmured something about not caring one way or the other, because I was afraid my appetites would get the best of me, that they would expose my wild and powerful hunger." She vocalizes what is true for so many of us. A fear of our own hunger and what it will do to us if we attempt to satiate it.

2. It makes us feel better. Looking at our growing credit card bill and shrinking paycheck feels…well, uncomfortable. I have turned to food to feel better on many occasions. The relief was brief, and the consequences only added to my discomfort in the long-term.

3. It's what everyone else is doing. I don't want to be the nerd at the party who isn't enjoying the social snacking and drinking. That's…uncomfortable. I'm not fitting in if I don't serve food or eat the food I'm served at every social engagement. Also, it might be yummy. I don't want the pain of knowing I've missed something delicious.

And so, we bow to our master and destroy our lives with every hasty *yes*.

I can't help but think of Augustus, Violet, Veruca, and Mike who tour Willy Wonka's chocolate factory with Charlie. Coming from a loving home with little money, Charlie has learned to wait for the good things in life. He has *had* to. But where scarcity reigned, love reigned greater, and he was able to develop the discipline of waiting. Of delaying. Unfortunately, his tour-mates, all of whom came from more affluence and privilege, had *not* learned the discipline of waiting. Their wants had never been delayed.

Wonka wanted an heir and thus made it possible for five "winners" with the golden tickets to tour his factory and, unbeknownst to them, also be tested in character. Author Roald Dahl ensured that each of the other characters dealt with a kind of vice, whether it was greed with food, demanding every want, obsession with television, or boastful and competitive. Ultimately, each of Charlie's tour-mates eliminate themselves by acting on their vices. *By refusing to delay their gratification*, to say *no* to themselves in the short-term for the *unknown* but still available long-term gain. Augustus falls into the chocolate river while trying to drink from it, getting sucked into the pipelines. Violet snatches a gum-in-testing from the protesting Wonka and chews it…unfortunately, a side effect of the not-yet-released gum included ballooning up into a huge blueberry. She has to be rolled out of the room and juiced. Mike, again against the protests of Wonka, places himself within a shrinking machine (meant for chocolate to be given through television sets) and is shrunk to only inches tall. Then finally, Veruca, who wanted Wonka to sell her a trained squirrel and was *denied*, thus jumping into the room to take one for herself. The squirrels decide she's a "bad nut" and off she goes to the garbage chute.

Only Charlie, who not only passed every opportunity to indulge, but honored the warnings of Wonka, is awarded the *grand prize* of becoming heir of the chocolate factory.

Only Charlie had developed a discipline of waiting. And only Charlie saw the result of lesser *noes* for the best *yes*.

So how do we overthrow the master we've served for so long? How did we survive an entire year of *waiting* for what we needed, when it was available with a shiny label just around the corner? Well, we failed a time or two, which I'll share later. But for the most part, we had to change our mindset. We had to redefine pleasure. We had to be mindful of the messages any given item might be whispering to us. We had to let ourselves become comfortable with uncomfortable. And I had to think about the Marcy a year from now. Who did I want her to be? We needed the discipline of Charlie Bucket.

For example, the first few times we shopped for groceries, we had to pull things *out of the cart.* Things that weren't food, but simple impulse-buys we mindlessly added. A magazine. A toy for one of our kids. A water game for the yard. A discounted movie. To develop a discipline of waiting, we had to actually put waiting into practice. We pulled the things out of the cart and put them back on the shelf. Over and over. Until one day, we didn't put it in the cart to begin with. We'd developed a discipline muscle. We were getting stronger.

We had to redefine "pleasure." For some, pleasure brings status. Stuff equals status which equals pleasure. A new car or brand clothing, the right-label purse, might communicate to my peers that I'm a person of affluence, and thus, worthy of love and affection and acceptance. For some, there's a transcendent pleasure—a pleasure that's not found in *stuff,* like meditation or prayer, silence, living healthy, listening to or performing music, etc. For others, the *anticipation* can *be* the pleasure. Redefining pleasure requires addressing the messages you hear with the decisions you make. Will buying this item give me something emotional? Societal? Physical? Is the promise it's making *true*? Is it what I want in the short-term *and* the long-term?

This meant that I had to stop and think of my future self, too. Would Marcy-of-tomorrow be proud of me today for making this decision? Would she be angry with me? Disappointed? Am I serving her *now* by giving into this message, buying the thing? Marcy-of-today learned that there's *so* much value in waiting. And one way I can love the Marcy-of-tomorrow is by really being clear on whether the waiting serves me or doesn't.

In the 1960's, there was a well-known study done known as the Marshmallow Experiment. Researchers gave four- and five-year old kids a marshmallow. The kids were told that if they waited fifteen minutes without eating the marshmallow, they'd receive a second marshmallow. The researcher then left the room for the child to be alone with their marshmallow. Eat one now or get two in fifteen minutes. Naturally, some kids gulfed their marshmallow immediately. Some wiggled and tried…but ended up eating it before the time expired. And a handful of kids made it to the end, receiving their much-anticipated reward.

The researchers followed the four- and five-year-old kids for over forty years and made a surprising discovery. In a discussion of the findings, James

Clear says, "The children who were willing to delay gratification and waited to receive the second marshmallow ended up having higher SAT scores, lower levels of substance abuse, lower likelihood of obesity, better responses to stress, better social skills as reported by their parents, and generally better scores in a range of other life measures. The researchers followed each child for more than forty years and over and over again, the group who waited patiently for the second marshmallow succeeded in whatever capacity they were measuring. In other words, this series of experiments proved that the ability to delay gratification was critical for success in life."[5]

Follow up studies further revealed that kids who'd had an opportunity to develop a level of *trust* that waiting would lead to a reward, were more likely to delay gratification. Saying a lesser no for a better yes wasn't a skill they were born with. It was a skill they developed. They'd had opportunities in their homes, already by the ages of four and five, to *learn the rewards of waiting*. There are many adults who haven't learned this yet! And honestly, we were among them in some ways! Still living as babies, filling every craving before it turned into discomfort or pain.

Yet the priceless rewards of waiting are immediate *and* lifelong. By telling ourselves *no* and choosing to wait, we have a chance to develop self-control. This means that larger life decisions are made with more wisdom and thoughtfulness because we aren't pressured by our craving for a quick yes. We can think it through because we are becoming the masters of our own decisions.

In our process of learning to wait, we developed appreciation. Man, did I come to truly treasure the items I found that met a need or desire in my heart. I earlier shared the story of finding an immersion blender I had really wanted and tried—oh so patiently—to find used (Blog Post—June—Immersion Blender FREEBIE). Let me tell you, ten years later, I still can't look at an immersion blender without a deep sense of gratitude and appreciation!

We developed a tolerance for pain and discomfort. Our resiliency grew. Our waiting didn't end when our experiment ended. Life is *full* of seasons of waiting. Waiting for a move. A new job. A raise. News on the health of a friend. Healing when that friend dies too young. Adoptions to finalize. An important piece of mail to arrive. The verdict. So. Much. Waiting. Because we'd forced ourselves to practice the *wait*, we grew in our ability to do so without panic, fear, and anxiety. Like the kids in the Marshmallow Experiment, we'd given ourselves an opportunity to experience firsthand the rewards of waiting. And with each reward, our ability to wait, to say slow yeses and necessary noes, became an act of anticipation rather than fret.

Consider book publishing. According to author Joseph Epstein, eighty-one percent of Americans want to write a book. Yet between one and two percent actually do it. There are a variety of reasons for this, but as an Author Success Coach who *gives writers all the tools for writing and publishing*, I see people quit all of the time. I even had one client say, "I'm not willing to make any more sacrifices to make this book happen. I've made enough as it is." He was done waiting. Couldn't be bothered to think of his future self, holding that published book, reading reviews from impacted readers, to keep moving forward. This is so common. People quitting on their dreams because they're *hard*. They make us uncomfortable. We feel pain. Writing and publishing is full of pain and discomfort! All of which feeds into the most beautiful character development and transformation—and I get to see it firsthand on a daily basis. If only the other 79-80% could wait for the second marshmallow, what a treat they'd get!

So how do we start? How do we face our fear of pain and discomfort so we're no longer mastered by the giant? Jonathan Bricker's TEDx Talk titled, *The Secret to Self-Control* has over five million views. Why? Because over five million people lack self-control but want it! In his talk, Bricker shares his epiphany that we must *feel* the feelings of our wants and needs in order to *overcome* them. Avoiding tends to trigger a greater desire *for* the object of our avoidance. But acknowledging the pain and the discomfort actually creates space in us to not need it. He covers exceptions to this, but for the most part, facing our pain disempowers it and gives the power back to us.

Who knew how *waiting* would be such a powerful teacher in my life? I had no idea that January how much waiting was ahead of me, and how much joy it would ultimately bring. The relationships I'd form. The items I'd receive. The items I'd give to the exact right person at the exact right time. I'm so glad the Marcy-of-2010 was willing to face pain head-on, because I've seen a *great deal of pain* ever since and she equipped me. She gave me experiences with waiting in safe spaces for me to develop the discipline that would later save my life and my marriage. She taught me that I can survive delayed gratification. And she taught me that often, when I wait, something better is around the corner.

Waiting is a powerful gift, if we can handle it. But we can also put our lives on hold and call it "waiting." Let's take a look at the difference in the next chapter.

[1] Johnson, A. (2013, June 24). 76% of Americans are living paycheck-to-paycheck. Retrieved May 17, 2020, from https://money.cnn.com/2013/06/24/pf/emergency-savings/

[2] Fay, B. (2019, December 05). Consumer Debt Statistics & Demographics in America. Retrieved May 19, 2020, from https://www.debt.org/faqs/americans-in-debt/demographics/

[3] Fay, B. (2019, November 07). The U.S. Consumer Debt Crisis. Retrieved May 19, 2020, from https://www.debt.org/faqs/americans-in-debt/

[4] Galvin, G. (2020, February 27). America Has Gotten Much Fatter in the Past Two Decades. Retrieved May 19, 2020, from https://www.usnews.com/news/healthiest-communities/articles/2020-02-27/us-obesity-rate-passes-40-percent

[5] Clear, J. (2020, February 04). The Marshmallow Experiment and the Power of Delayed Gratification. Retrieved May 19, 2020, from https://jamesclear.com/delayed-gratification

Blog Post—January—Why Wait?

We had an appointment with our financial adviser, Michael Burton, the other day. He works for Everance Financial Advisors. It's a free service and he's also a dear friend of ours from college.

I remember the first time I walked into his office. It was Jeremy's idea and I was mortified. I felt like I was walking in totally nude as we laid bare our finances before his scrutiny. It ends up that God has called him to his role in finances and he has not been our judge or enemy. But I'm sure you know the feeling. I know you feel the heat rise and the heart rate increase when you think of someone looking at *every* penny you spend wondering at all the things they might suggest cutting out. Well, that's not what he does. He has helped us get rid of all of our debt and to continue to live debt free, with good sound advice on purchases (when we seek his council, which we do often) and life insurance policies, living trusts, etc. And, Everance is a faith-based organization so it's all with godly stewardship in mind. We still get to eat out, buy things, take trips, watch movies, etc.

Anyway, we had a meeting with him and shared our resolution for the year, which, funny enough, didn't save us any money this month. We still ran out. Of course, I did go to New York.

Anyway (focus, Marcy), I would like braces. We would like a repaired fence. I "need" a sewing machine—so many "things." We happen to have a source of set-aside money that we can pull from and we periodically dip into it.

During this visit, Michael kept asking, "Is that something you can save up for?" *silence*

"Well, yeah, I guess we could." Save up for things? Who does that anymore?

We live in such a culture of immediate gratification. If I want something, I go buy it. And then I buy something extra just because I can. There's no waiting. No delay. Our national mentality (even in government) seems to be, "Why save for what you can buy with credit today?" I hadn't even considered that as being part of my *family* culture. We don't have debt. We don't charge things. We don't finance things (except our house). But we do dip into savings. Jeremy's Master's program, my continued education classes, small road trips...

This has really got me thinking. The best things in life are the things you have to wait for: A spouse, children, a much-needed vacation, fruit fresh off the tree in their seasons—some things can't be rushed.

My last journal entry was on the blessing we might *lose* when we meet our own needs. This one is on the blessings we lose when we won't wait for them from God's hand. Really, I've lived twenty-nine years with these teeth. What's another year of saving up for braces? Had I rushed out and bought a new sewing machine, I wouldn't have the gift of the one loaned to me (that I get to give some life to for its owner). I find that I can *truly* appreciate something if it took some effort to get it. I have a new appreciation for paper. I have a new appreciation for fireplace keys, sewing machines, dressers, my community.

Proverbs 8:34

Blessed is the man who listens to me, watching daily at my doors, waiting at my doorway.

Isaiah 30:18

Yet the LORD longs to be gracious to you; He rises to show you compassion. For the LORD is a God of justice. Blessed are all who wait for Him!

Isaiah 64:4

Since ancient times no one has heard, no ear has perceived, no eye has seen any God besides you, who acts on behalf of those who wait for Him.

We will begin saving for the things (even used ones) that we want/need. Greater, we will be waiting on the Lord to meet those needs and desires as He pleases! May we all learn the patience that leads to His blessing.

Chapter 9

Living on Your Own Excess

Now that we've talked a minute about the value of waiting, let's also discuss how to misuse it. Waiting can get *in the way*. That's right. We can defer our lives by always waiting for it to get better. This is *not* the waiting I was talking about in the last chapter. This is putting off your life in the hopes that the next new shiny object will finally be the thing that makes you feel whole. And as we pursue each new item, we end up with homes and hearts overflowing with low quality excess.

What if what I have isn't enough? What if I allow myself to feel satisfied with the contents within my walls, and then I miss the life satisfaction the next thing would have brought? We live in a constant *stuff* FOMO. What if I don't upgrade my phone to the newest, fastest, most capable version available and my pictures are less quality than they *could* be? Unlimited data? Isn't that what I need for happiness and fulfillment? We withhold from ourselves the joy of *now* by anticipating the next unknown trinket that will finally settle our souls. All the while, we surround ourselves with more and more, until it overflows into our garages, sheds, and storage units.

Yet has *more* really ever improved the quality of your life? I suppose I can think of an item or two that brought sincere pleasure…for a minute. Or maybe years. But most of the stuff *around it* was clutter. And the *reason* it brought pleasure may have been misguided. Before moving to Germany, I had a plethora of Pepsi bottles that I had collected from around the world. It was my token souvenir. As airlines tightened up policies around liquids, I had to get creative about how to get my prized possessions home, to sit on my shelf and proudly display my travel prowess. I mean, isn't that why they brought me such joy? Deep down, they said, "You are valuable, Marcy. Look at all the places you've been. People will see that and finally see how worthy you are of attention and affection." Of course, I didn't stop to really *listen* to the message. I just agreed with it and started up a dusty collection of useless cans and bottles. Sure, friends saw them and thought I was cool. Or weird. But when I was confronted with a cross-global move, I had to make a decision about these cans and bottles. Was I really going to *pay* to fly them across the world to my new home?

No. I was not. So instead, I took pictures to remember my quirky habit and recycled the cans and bottles. Have I missed them a second since? Nope. Now when I'm traveling, I find a Pepsi, I drink it and savor the moment I'm given, and move on. Now, I realize I made this sound really *easy*. It wasn't. Letting go of the items that ascribed some level of value to my identity was painful. Realizing that I had allowed tin and plastic to ascribe value to me was even worse. Embarrassing and shameful. But this was after our year of not buying new things and I had developed a discipline of facing my pain, acknowledging the feelings, and letting go.

This is why the Marie Kondo phenomenon has been so powerful. The KonMarie premise is to "keep only those things that speak to your heart. Then take the plunge and discard all the rest." Well, my cans and bottles spoke to my heart, all right, but not in a way that supported the truth of my identity and value. Marie goes on to say, "No matter how wonderful things used to be, we cannot live in the past. The joy and excitement we feel here and now are more important." We must choose to *stop waiting* for the next shiny object that will magically solve all that feels empty in us and live *now*. Live well with what we already have.

There is a cost, a heavy burden, to living with so much excess (and regularly adding to it). That cost isn't just financial.

Neuroscientists at Princeton University found that stuff actually competes for our attention, increasing stress and reducing your productivity. Yes! Living with excess, even if it's just lying around taking up space, makes you less productive. Your brain can't fully focus on the things that truly give you joy, or an income, when it's competing with categorizing the messages of such a large amount of stuff.

It gets worse. Researchers at UCLA studied a number of families and found that *every single mother's* stress levels spiked when she was dealing with their belongings. As if raising children, marriage, and household management didn't create enough of its own stress. We certainly don't need mothers with more of the stress hormone Cortisol coursing through their systems. While helpful for survival, it's *not* helpful for utilizing the parts of our brain that we need for goal setting, cause-and-effect thinking, prioritizing, critical thinking, or even using the language centers of our brain. (Ever find your words coming out jumbled or forgetting them altogether? Stress can have that effect!)

I've also heard it said that some people (and I'm sure I'm one of them) can *hear* stuff. That when they walk into a room and see clutter or excess, it presents as noise in their heads. This resonated deeply with me. If I walk into a disorganized, over-flowing space of stuff, you might as well be banging pots in my ears. I'm so distracted by my discomfort that I can't hear someone speaking to me. When the stuff is out of control, I can only turn and walk out of the room, leaving the mess shouting at my back as I retreat. Refusing to add to my excess (and address the excess I already have) actually quiets my space so I can sit and enjoy it peacefully.

If this noise isn't shouting at me, increasing my Cortisol, or making me all around less productive, then it's still having an immediate impact on my life through the planet I live on. Since I can't *leave* earth as a normal, living, not-employed-by-NASA person, the impact on the earth is impact on *me*. And you better believe that our over-indulgence in stuff has affected the earth. In a fascinating article called *Excessive Consumption—America's Real Addiction*, the author says, "Should we fail to reconcile voluntarily the 'infiniteness' associated with our material wants and expectations with the 'finiteness' associated with the earth's natural resources and derivative economic resources—thereby remaining addicted to excessive consumption—we will reach one or more limits. That is, either the sources of our ecological and economic indiscretions will no longer be willing or able to support our continued profligacy, or the consequences associated with our indiscretions will simply overwhelm us."[1] Basically, if we don't get a hold of our excessive lifestyles, we're going to destroy the planet, and in doing so, our own happiness. We strive for the short-term pleasure, missing that we're killing our end-goal the whole time.

There are so many conversations on the topic of saving the earth, so I'll spare you any depths of it here. The point to take home is that the clutter in our homes doesn't only impact *us*. It impacts the planet and everyone we share it with. In 1994, delegates to the Cairo International Conference on Population and Development were alarmed to learn that *one baby born in the US* will consume twenty times more of the world's resources than a child born in Africa or India. Where some had argued that overpopulation is the planet's problem, representatives from developing countries advocated that the problem is *overconsumption in the North*.[2] My clutter and your stuff feeds the statistic. We have power to say, "No more."

We've been asking the right question but satisfied with the wrong answer. The question hasn't been, "Will this make me happy?" or even "Do I need this?" The underlying question to our inordinate consumption is "Am I enough?" Am I worthy of love and affection? Am I special? Am I valuable? Am I *enough* to warrant love and affection, uniqueness, and value? This is a terribly important question and we've been satisfied with a lie for an answer. Marketing teams have known for a long time that this is your deep unresolved question. They scheme at ways to poke at the pain of this unanswered mystery, willing to fill in the empty spaces with their newest, brightest service or package. And we've fallen for it. We fell for the lie that the fidget spinner would make us the cool kid and we'd have the promise of admiring friends for life if we could just own *ten*. Or that the car with the sunroof and DVD players behind the headrests would finally make us the family we've always dreamed of being. That the envy of our friends and family and neighbors would finally prove that we've *arrived*.

The answer, friend, is far simpler than they've led you to believe.

Yes.

The answer is YES. You *are* worthy of love and affection, of the uniqueness that makes you shine, and of the value you behold. Yes. You don't need to believe it to make it true. You don't need to buy the next promise to make it real. You just *are*. Not every broken person sharing this space with you will validate that, see it, affirm it, or honor it. Because they're asking the *same* question and looking for answers in all the ways, even the ways that mean tearing you down for their own security. (We'll cover that in the next chapter).

YES.

So now that you know the answer to your deepest question, what can you gain from living on what you already have? What is the *gain* of less? It's still not your value, your worthiness, your uniqueness. You've already got that. The gains are cherries on an already beautiful cake.

Imagine what we could do with the money we're *not* spending on more stuff? Have you had a dream to see the world? You can. Have you seen poverty and hardship in the world and thought, *What can I do to change that?* You can change it. Have you wanted to impact lives? Take a writing or speaking course. Have you wanted to contribute to humanitarian work or disaster relief? Support a missionary or a relief-response organization.

Imagine how your money, or even your *stuff*, might have meaning bigger and brighter than your own wallet and shelf. How maybe you're holding back, getting in the way even, of the gift you could give our global community if you could know you're loved and share your excess with others. Wow! It's powerful. Harvey Mackay once said, "If you can afford a fancy car, you can make more of an impact driving an ordinary one." You have the power to change the world, starting with living with what you already have and being a good steward of it.

Imagine the creativity you would engage to live with what you already have? The creativity to recycle, upcycle, and repurpose the things sitting in your own corners. We have supported (and even served alongside) a wonderful organization called HaitiGo as they offer community development to rural regions of Haiti. One of the programs that I *love* has come alongside the women of these areas and taught them how to turn cereal boxes into gorgeous pieces of jewelry through the Haitian Bead Project. They themselves didn't have an over-abundance of cereal boxes like we do, so as a local community we saved and stored away our boxes to send to Haiti. The jewelry that comes back is unexplainable. The way they use the colors and the text to create *an income source* for their family is incredible. I witnessed how an excess of my nation (what we would consider trash) could be repurposed into something beyond my imagination.

When waves of refugees hit Germany, with over a million people looking for asylum, I worked in the camps. We didn't share a language, but we shared living as foreigners and strangers in a place not where we were raised. With time, I was able to develop deep relationships with the women and their families. We brought the Cereal-box-jewelry-project to the ladies and kids one day. Yep, Germany has an excess of printed cardboard too. We taught them how to roll the beads with glue and sticks and create necklaces, lanyards, earrings, keychains, you name it. We shared smiles, laughter, and awe at the skill with which these new friends could, again, repurpose what most consider garbage. This is only one example of how one person's trash can be another person's income stream. Other examples include the bracelets and messenger bags that have been made from the life vests strewn about from refugees crossing from Turkey to Greece, or rain boots turned plant holders, ladders turned into living room decor, tires turned into playground equipment. Just search "repurpose ideas" on the Internet and you'll find over *twenty-four million* creative ways to take what you have and use it for something new (or release it to be used as something new by someone else!). Yes, living with what we have engages our creativity.

Speaking of engaging your creativity, did you know that researchers have found "that people who engaged in artistic activities, such as painting, drawing and sculpting, in both middle and old age were 73% less likely to have memory and thinking problems, such as mild cognitive impairment, that lead to dementia. The study also revealed that craft-based activities such as sewing, woodworking and ceramics in midlife and old age, were 45% less likely to encounter cognitive issues."[3] That's right, folks. Utilizing your creative center has actually shown less likelihood of Dementia and Alzheimer's. What do you have to gain by repurposing what you have? Oh, just your quality of life in your final years.

But not only are the gains for your future self, they involve your current self, too. If you *know* your worth is yours, outside of what you own, you can stop deferring your life and live in the present. You can enjoy *now*. You can be content with what you have right in front of you. "We tend to forget that happiness doesn't come as a result of getting something we don't have, but rather of recognizing and appreciating what we do have" (Frederick Keonig). Being present means you have peace of mind, you don't *miss* the joys right in front of you, actually *living* your life instead of waiting for it to begin.

Being present can feel painful. It's not easy. Marie Kondo says, "The process of facing and selecting our possessions can be quite painful. It forces us to confront our imperfections and inadequacies and the foolish choices we made in the past." Being present means *feeling presently*. And sometimes what we feel isn't pretty. But sometimes what we feel isn't based on the truth, either. Or if it is, then we get to choose to empower ourselves to overcome those feelings. For example, did you know that your brain can*not* experience both worry and gratitude at the same time? Both of those are feelings, and they don't mesh. But *you* have the choice, the power to decide which one you want to experience. Stress and contentment exist in two different parts of the brain, and they fight for the blood flow. The more blood flowing, the more oxygen moving, the more you'll experience the feeling. This happens with or without your conscious effort. But, when you *add* your conscious effort, you can effect change! Here's what I mean.

Say I'm stressed about taxes (totally hypothetical!). I open the tax bill and my brain interprets the number listed. The number I'm supposed to write on a check and send off to Uncle Sam. Immediately, my instinctual response might be Fight or Flight. Survive. *Stress.*

- I can ignore it (put off paying the bill and prioritize it waaaaay low on the list of priorities).
- I can feel it and frenzy over it (mull over all of the "what if" questions. What if I need that money? What if they made a mistake? What if I end up broke on the street? How will I feed my family?).
- I can reframe it: Wow, I made enough money this year that I owe taxes? What a gift to be able to provide for my family and *now* for my country too. What a gift to live in a country that allows me to pursue my dreams and make an income at the same time.

When you choose either of the first two options, you're letting your brain take its natural course. But when you choose option three, you're utilizing your power to combat *nature*. You are grabbing your end of the tug-of-war rope and demanding to be *heard*. You are no longer a slave to your natural processes and now in control of your neurological system, which you *can* be! When you choose to reframe your experience, you're showing your brain that this isn't Flight or Fight at all. That you are *safe*. And you are! When you choose gratitude, you force the blood flow away from stress, negativity, and anxiety and *toward* gratitude, contentment, and peace. It's not easy at first. It's really is a tug of war so you have to TUG. Choose to speak out the gifts you find in the surprise obstacle and, before you know it, your blood flow will switch directions and you'll feel a new ease in seeing the positive picture. You have to fight for it. It's worth fighting for. Choose gratitude and you *cannot* feel the stress.

A verse in the Bible that I aim for as a lifestyle, by engaging the above battle, is spoken by Paul, a man who murdered those who followed Jesus before having an incredible encounter with the resurrected Jesus. He says, *"I know what it is to be in need, and I know what it is to have plenty. I have learned the secret of being content in any and every situation, whether well-fed or hungry, whether living in plenty or in want"* (Philippians 4:12). He only got there by submitting his feelings to a higher power, to a source of gratitude regardless of circumstance. He wrote this from prison. Training ourselves into true contentment is a *huge gain* when we choose to live on what we already have.

As we choose to live on less, or live on what we already have, we experience less stress. We will spend less money, freeing up our bank accounts for things that really matter. We begin to live high-quality lives with less low-quality junk. And we are immediately free of the pressure to keep up with the Joneses. Can you imagine appreciating what you already have? You could watch your neighbor add on a guest house suite to their house and not have to entertain a single thought about how you'll be able to afford to keep up with their appearances. You can look around your space and love what you see, the people you see in it, and the life unfolding in all its simple glory.

What would living with what you already have mean for you? What has it meant for you, really, to live with so much excess in your life? When you reflect on this chapter, imagine yourself in the following two scenarios.

You look around and there's stuff everywhere. Someone made lunch and left out their trash. A sock is on the floor, not terribly far from a discarded grocery bag and a popsicle stick. Dust coats picture frames and doodads decorating open spaces on shelves. A pile of belongings sits at the base of the stairs, waiting for their owner to carry them up and put them away. The laundry overflows like a volcanic eruption on the couch. The bookshelves are lined with books, board games, and that sweet figurine collection you've accrued by your favorite artist. If you're like me, then in this scenario you'll immediately feel a weight on your chest just thinking about it. The noise of your stuff picks up the volume. Your breathing feels tight, and no, it's not asthma. It's the weight of even the *idea* of so much stuff.

Now imagine yourself in this second scenario. You've battled the bloodflow in your brain, and you feel contentment and peace. You look around and are satisfied. Your creativity is flowing. Your relationships flourishing. Your bank account busting. What would it mean for you to live like this? Take some time to reflect on this and journal it somewhere.

Now, what's stopping you? What's in the way of you choosing scenario two? No one is saying it's easy, even if it feels amazing. Getting started with any change in life is *hard*. But guess what? You have a history of overcoming hard things. It's made you stronger than you realize. So, what's in the way of living peacefully with what you already have? Take some time to process that and jot it down, too.

You see, when we name things, we strip them of their power. This beast that's been threatening to destroy you if you even *try* to improve your quality of life…well, it's actually only a peanut. A peanut with a teeny, screechy voice that's been playing shadow games with you. Make some peanut butter and be on your way.

There are a number of ways to live with what you already have. Addressing the above questions will make the following so much easier. Acknowledging and correcting any limiting beliefs about your value and status will release a flow of peace and creativity. Have an old cookie pan lying around? Get rid of it or google "repurposing a cookie pan." Let your creativity flow. Or let someone else's flow and donate it. Say goodbye to it. Kondo says, "The process of assessing how you feel about the things you own, identifying those that have fulfilled their purpose, expressing your gratitude, and bidding them farewell is really about examining your inner self, a rite of passage to a new life." Whether it stays or goes, make sure it's taking up only the amount of space you give it. And make peace with it.

And while you're at it, make peace with the folks who can't understand *why in the world* you would do anything like this! In the next chapter, we'll talk about the responses we got to our decision to buy used for a year, and how to make peace with differing opinions around your healthy life choices.

---

[1] Clugston, C. (2007, October 20). Excessive Consumption—America's Real Addiction. Retrieved May 20, 2020, from http://www.culturechange.org/cms/content/view/128/1/

[2] Sagoff, M. (2014, September 26). Do We Consume Too Much? Retrieved May 20, 2020, from https://www.theatlantic.com/magazine/archive/1997/06/do-we-consume-too-much/376877/

[3] Strickland, A. (2015, April 09). Could creativity and socializing preserve your memory? Retrieved May 20, 2020, from https://edition.cnn.com/2015/04/09/health/creativity-socializing-delay-dementia/index.html

Blog Post—January—Moochers

I have noticed an interesting phenomenon over the last twenty days of our resolution.

First: I often feel the need to explain that I'm not just *taking* from the community, but that I'm also giving. Some people respond with thrill when we describe our goal, some even feel inspired to join us in some form or another. Others seem to have a "so you're gonna mooch on society" type attitude. This has been rare but not absent.

Second: I often notice others feel the need to defend their own use of "Freecycle" or the idea of re-using other people's items. Now, I *know* that I'm not standing in judgment of them so it's not my subtle attitude causing them to give me an explanation.

These two things have caused me a lot of pondering. Why would we feel embarrassed, defensive, judged, for choosing to live within a community that shares its excess? This makes me sad. I don't have the answers now. I can imagine that the few people who've taken advantage of the generosity of others has given *all* recyclers fear of being viewed as the same. This is unfortunate.

Acts 2:45-47 says, "All the believers were together and had everything in common. Selling their possessions and goods, they gave to anyone as he had need. Every day they continued to meet together in the temple courts. They broke bread in their homes and ate together with glad and sincere hearts, praising God and enjoying the favor of all the people. And the Lord added to their number daily those who were being saved."

What an awesome vision for this life of living on excess! *This* is my vision—not to spend as little money as possible by taking from others, but to support *all* who are in need, and to be supported. There was no shame in this. Only joy.

May we each find the joy as we are blessed with the "extra" others give as well as the joy found in giving our "extra" to others. Give to everyone who has a need, no matter how big or small, and see how

God meets your *own* needs, sometimes through others, sometimes through sheer miracles, sometimes through freecycling.

I will end on this note. I will not defend our choice by listing all of the things I have given away, as if to justify asking for things I need. Just as I will not ask for a list of donations from a brother or sister in need to whom I am giving my things. In a world *so* focused on self-interests and self-gain, we will certainly come across people who just don't understand. May we seek only to please our Lord and be justified before Him as we make decisions based on prayer and Scripture in an effort to live Spirit-filled lives. Go, therefore, give and receive!

Chapter 10
Dealing with Embarrassment

One of the things that caught me totally off-guard were a few people who couldn't or wouldn't understand what we were doing. They'd make comments, even calling us names (you know, in that friendly but pointed social media kind of way). Moochers. How dare we try to live off the backs of other people's labor?! They were definitely the minority, but negative voices like that sure seem to overpower the positive, affirming ones, don't they?

They rattled me a bit. Was I really attempting to live off the hard work of others for a year? Was I just trying to "mooch" off the excess of others for my own gain? I'd try to explain our purpose but to no avail. These people just refused to buy into our plan to create community, reduce national excess (starting with our own home and habits), and see what would happen in the process.

So, I tried to sit and be a good listener. To understand what so unsettled them about our own little personal journey buying used for a year. I tried to listen beneath the names and accusations and straight into the heart of the messages that these people were operating from.

Brené Brown says, "You can choose courage, or you can choose comfort, but you cannot choose both." I didn't expect to need courage in facing a few of our relationships. I expected to need courage in the actual *doing* of the experiment, but not in explaining it to people. But as Dieter Uchtdorf says, "It is your reaction to adversity, not the adversity itself, that determines how your life's story will develop." I knew that digging in with these folks would help me further solidify and understand our purposes going into this year. Maybe we *were* moochers! I wouldn't know if I didn't really sit with the possibilities, investigate them, make decisions about them, and move forward.

I love what Shauna Niequist says in her book, *Bread and Wine*. "One thing's for sure: if you decide to be courageous and sane, if you decide not to overspend or overcommit or overschedule, the healthy people in your life will respect those choices. And the unhealthy people in your life will freak out, because you're making a healthy choice they're not currently free to make. Don't for one second let that stop you."

Ultimately, I determined that we were not trying to be the leeches of society, but the exact opposite. To stop being dependent on marketing messages for our definition of "value" and pave a new path in *our* home for living well, healthy, and in solidarity with people around us. Even the ones who disagreed or didn't get it.

If, as Coco Chanel said, "The most courageous act is still to think for yourself. Aloud," then my job was to keep being open to the conversation but willing to come to my own, different conclusions. Out loud. So, I blogged. I shared. I processed. I practiced courage. And I learned a few things about myself and others in the process.

There are a number of reasons, I realized, why people might respond poorly. And by "poorly," I specifically mean being unable to understand or straight rejecting our purpose for buying used items for a year and responding unkindly.

1. Guilt—sometimes the success of another person pricks our own conscience. Sometimes changes, even good ones, make us evaluate our own lives and feel uncomfortable. Maybe *I* should be doing something about that as well…

2. Threat to Status Quo—Sometimes when we make positive changes in our lives, our endeavor rubs up against the status quo. It suddenly raises the bar for what has otherwise been an understood way of doing things. This can feel threatening to people who are comfortable and fear being uncomfortable.

3. Insecurity—Truly secure people can allow others to change without it impacting who *they* are. But insecure people, those who are still looking for their value in external things, feel rocked and rattled when something in their atmosphere shifts. If you're shifting, prepare for some words. They're afraid.

4. Fear of Losing the Relationship—I've heard of this in new marriages. A sibling or parent fears they will lose the relationship once their loved one enters matrimony. Our relationships matter. They're significant and often a large source of where we find our value. When the relationship feels threatened, people go sour. Sometimes, even when you choose to buy used things for a year, people worry that you'll change too much, changing the relationship as they've known it as you go along.

5. Our Pain, Their Gain—Have you ever heard of the DUFF? The Designated Ugly Fat Friend. Yep, and everybody wants one. Studies have shown how having a DUFF actually elevates the *perceived attractiveness* in others around them. "Research published in the journal *Psychological Science* has shown that judgements of attractiveness vary depending on who is nearby, and how good-looking they are in comparison. A person will rank higher on a scale of attractiveness when compared alongside less attractive people, than they would when judged alone."[1] Sometimes, keeping others "beneath" them somehow protects their fragile sense of self. Change who you are, and you change who *they* are.

6. Envy—Sometimes a shift in your life is also a shift in your social status. Or at least, the perception of your social status. You'll become more "privileged" and sometimes, people around you make upward social comparisons. It was fine while you were rubbing shoulders in the same social stratosphere but if *you* elevate, what does that mean for them?

7. Haters Gonna Hate—Sometimes people live critical lives. For whatever reason, the cynical monster has climbed right up into their brains and taken up residence. No matter what good comes their way, they'll only see a reason to complain. But the reality is what Marie Kondo says, "To get rid of what you no longer need is neither wasteful nor shameful." They can whine and poo-poo but making positive changes are just that—positive.

8. Huh?—Sometimes, they just literally don't understand. They have had different life experiences, different values, different upbringing, different awareness, different Enneagram number, different *you-name-it*. And try as you might, they legit cannot understand what you're doing or why. And understanding matters to them. They can't let it go until they understand…but they won't. And that's okay.

Feeling judged? Misunderstood? You're in good company. Feeling misunderstood is a major pet peeve of mine. I bet if you added all the hours I've spent explaining myself to people to overcome my own discomfort of being misunderstood, those hours could circle the moon fifty-nine times. I'm not really sure how many hours that makes but it seems like a lot. I've had to learn to let it go. Yep, just like Elsa.

But you know what? The baggage of other people is no reason for us to stay the same. In fact, their discomfort can strengthen us. Mahatma Gandhi said, "Strength does not come from winning. Your struggles develop your strengths. When you go through hardships and decide not to surrender, that is strength." There were hardships in our experiment, and there were hardships in how the minority responded. But those hardships served to strengthen our resolve, encouraged us to self-evaluate, and reminded us the importance of trying new things. It's not for the pleasure of others, but to live according to our own conscience.

So, we did it anyway. It's what we knew was right for us. We wanted a better quality of life. We wanted our neighbors and community to have better qualities of life. Our whole world. But we had to start in our own home. Our pain should not be their crutch. Our response to the burden of our stuff didn't belong to anyone else's happiness. If living our best lives was threatening to a few, then I could recognize their place in their own journey, bless them, and move on.

And you should too. I don't mean spending a whole year refusing to buy new things, though that would be awesome. But you should rattle the status quo. Raise the bar. Is it terrible if people start to look at their own lives and feel uncomfortable? No way! It's the discomfort that often prompts us to *do something* about it. And who knows but maybe you'll convert a few of those skeptics years down the line, just because you didn't give in or give up when their words were against you. "Good timber does not grow with ease. The stronger the wind the stronger the trees" (Thomas S. Monson).

Here are some steps for preparing for your own life change, whatever it might be. Even baby steps toward health and wholeness need some preparation in place.

- Find a Supportive Community—Just like you'll find the naysayers, you'll find the people who've been waiting for the nudge to live for quality versus quantity.
- Set Small, Achievable Goals—Okay, maybe we're not the best role models for this by starting with an entire year as our social experiment timeframe. For us, it was perfect. But maybe you need to start smaller. Try a week. A holiday. A vacation. Or maybe it's not committing to used purchases and it's something entirely different. Give yourself a goal you can hit.
- Remind Yourself Why This Matters—When it starts to feel hard, when the waiting is smothering you, or when the messages are loud, it's easy to throw in the towel and quit. Instead, remind yourself why this is important to you! For us, we wanted to see *if it was possible* for a family like ours to live on used goods for a year. Quitting would leave that question unanswered. And it would mean missing unexpected opportunities with our local community.
- Give Them Space / Permission to Be Different—Expect people who struggle with your idea. That's okay. Give them space to have a different opinion. It's not a reflection of you, but of their own personal journey. And it's an important journey. Let them walk their road while respectfully sticking to yours.

I learned a lot from sharing about our experience. From the people who wanted to join us, to those who were inspired with a different but equally important idea, to those who struggled to make space for our resolution, I learned something. I learned to be strong. I learned to let go. And I learned to be gracious. Without contention or questioning, we'd be pansies.

Here's a word to you from Sir Anonymous, "Hang in there. Trust that those winds of adversity are blowing away what's not needed while making you stronger."

And we would *need* stronger. My sentimentalities were yet to be tested. With each holiday and tradition, I was tested in the winds of adversity, and boy was it windy! In the next chapter, I'll share how my sense of tradition and gift-giving was challenged.

---

[1] University of Royal Holloway London. (2016, September 29). Beauty of standing out in a crowd: Attractiveness judged according to who we are with, research shows. *ScienceDaily*. Retrieved May 20, 2020 from www.sciencedaily.com/releases/2016/09/160929082154.htm

Blog Post—January—Birthdays

Here's a thought. Perhaps you think that you will only be reading my story and not somehow involved. Wrong.

When your birthday or Christmas or Valentine's Day or *whatever* comes around, you will be getting a *used* gift from me. Don't be offended or surprised. At best, it will be homemade. At worst—it will be clearly used and re-gifted. Regardless, I love you.

HAPPY BIRTHDAY!

Blog Post—March—Celebrating Birthday Parties

I knew that when the birthdays of my children approached, I would have a harder time with this resolution. Up until now, we have had the delight and challenge of providing gifts for the individuals who have invited us to *their* parties. That was minor compared to planning a whole birthday party of things used, not to mention the gifts for my *own* child.

That said, I am thrilled to say that the birthday party *and* our resolution remained a compatible success of which I'm excited to share the journey.

The day was approaching quickly. I had posted a number of "wanted" and "looking for" ads in various Internet locations in the hopes of finding things to use for our son's room remodel. That is our gift to him—a newly painted and decorated bedroom to the theme of his heart's content. My daughter had hers done last March for her birthday. Fortunately, that means no other material gifts (and, as we found with my daughter, ends up being more expensive than if we just bought toys and wrapped them!). These two older children are my foster children who shall be adopted *any day now* (Lord willing) and so we are especially thrilled to do whatever we can to make this place *their* place.

That said, I was getting no response to my inquiries. All of a sudden it began to come together! I found a nearly new set of twin bedsheets, Superman themed, on Craigslist for five dollars! This was from a *very* nice and clean home and couldn't have been a better deal. I wouldn't have found that in a thrift store for that price.

In addition, a number of guests to his birthday party presented him with things to accent his room...hand painted Superman art, etc. Beautiful! Finally, I went into Salvation Army one day just to see what they had. I found still-new-in-wrapper streamers (one that actually said, "Happy Birthday" and the other solid red). Perfect! I also found a big bag of plastic Easter eggs, which is nice because I love to use these for Easter but had taken all of mine to Haiti last year when I taught our students how to make egg shakers. I also found a blue valance and red fabric to make a curtain.

All of that (plus some other little gems for myself) for only seven dollars. I'll be going back too, tons of Easter baskets, grass for baskets, etc. Ya know, they got used once and ended up at the thrift store. Perfect, I'll use them once more and send them back.

Needless to say, it was such a blessing to see friends, family, and thrift stores unite to make an amazing airplane-themed birthday party happen from scratch. We made paper airplanes (from the free legal sized paper I'd received) and had races. I made airplane favors out of Lifesavers, gum, and rubber bands and hung airline-themed signs all over the house. I *home-made* the ice cream cake (that was a first and lots of fun).

Another crazy gift—our church, The Bridge, is doing a series on Heroes. The designed backdrop of the series is a very large painting, of a cityscape. The amazing part is days before I found this out, my son told me how he wanted his room painted, you got it, with a cityscape. I thought I'd ask about getting the template from the church so I could use it for his room. Better yet, they offered to give me one of the paintings at the end of the series! What a "coincidence" (if I believe in coincidence) that would line these two events up at the same time and bless my son! Not to mention that I'm currently writing a book on humanity's search for a superhero...

My husband painted the cityscape on the wall. Some dear friends painted pictures to accent the walls. And we are waiting on one painting that we will get to add shortly. It was so neat to see it all come together. My son *loves* his room (as I'm sure you can imagine).

Having four kids means that I have three more birthday parties (plus my husband's) to plan with this same sort of creativity.

On a slightly separate note, I was putting together the kids' Easter baskets today. It struck me how much I was enjoying putting my creativity to use. Normally, I would have gone out and bought a couple baskets at Target or Walmart. Today I scoured my house for old but still nice gift bags. I found one that was Tinkerbell themed...perfect for my nine-year-old daughter. I found a solid red one that I added Superman stickers to for my oldest son. I had one bucket that I'd won from MOPS for my two-year-old son. And a blue gift bag with a boa accent (which I'd purchased at a thrift store) for my almost-one-year-old. I filled plastic eggs (thank you, Salvation Army) with candies and filled their little Easter bags. Anyway, I found myself enjoying creating these things for my children and putting to good use things I already owned. It will be a fun day, regardless!

Blog post—April—Another Birthday

Well, our New Year's resolution was tested yet again by another birthday! We celebrated my youngest love's first birthday! We decided to go Luau style since she wouldn't remember, and we would have lots of fun!

I was so blessed by the generosity of friends *and* our church to both loan and give us things for the Luau. *Every* decoration was provided for. My husband and youngest son had matching shirts (loaned to us) and my birthday baby had three Hawaiian dresses to pick from! She also had the cutest little grass skirt given to us. I found a couple leis at thrifts stores, but most were given or loaned to us. I offered leis as favors, but most people just left them. I made the cupcakes and we all barbecued. It was a really fun day. Instead of spending money on gifts for my birthday girl, we spent the money on loving our family and friends with a free meal. That was a definitely blessing. My daughter certainly won't remember that we didn't get her anything in particular...besides, so many others gave to her. We asked for used/re-used gifts so her birthday wouldn't cause *others* to buy new either. Some did, some didn't. But at the end of the day, I was so honored to spend the birthday money on our dear friends and family who so love my little one, instead of filling our house with a bunch of new, shiny, noisy imagination-killer toys.

Chapter 11

Birthdays and Holidays

While I was excited about our experiment to buy nothing new, I was pretty nervous about how that would work with holidays and traditions. You see, I'm pretty sentimental about these things. I *love* celebrating people and being celebrated. I love bringing close friends and family together in time-honored traditions.

Even though I was raised on welfare, my mom did an amazing job of making my sister and I feel loved. I'd sometimes come home to find some little memento on my bed, a treasure that reminded my mom of me while she was out running errands. Every little unnecessary gift said, "You matter when we're not together. I think of you because you're loved." This became how I understood love—as an actual, tangible, gift.

Maybe you've heard of *The Five Love Languages* by Gary Chapman. The premise is that each person receives and gives love in a particular way. And those ways are pretty distinct. For example, one of my top "love languages" is Gift-Giving. My husband's, however, is Acts of Service, with Gift-Giving way, way, way low on his list of languages. What does that mean? Disaster! Just kidding, it just means lots of therapy and two copies of *The Five Love Languages*. It also means that sometimes, I give him a gift to show my deep affection, and all he sees is another thing he'll have to dust. It quickly makes it to a pile of give-away items. I see my *love* in a box and am shattered. Well, that was before all of the therapy, anyway.

It also means that when he wants to show how much he loves me he does something for me. I mean, don't get me wrong, this is *really* nice. But it's also what I expect a partner in a household to do…share the load. He thinks he's scoring love points, and I see it as what he should do in honor of domestic equality. Come my birthday, when he doesn't have a thoughtful gift, I'm positive I'm in a loveless marriage. Come Christmas, if I give him a bunch of gifts, and neglect some way of supporting him through a service-oriented action, he might be wondering why we ever got married. (I did try last Christmas to get his bike repaired as his "gift." Unfortunately, my good intentions got as far as arranging with a friend to be the repair man. I told Jeremy my Christmas-gift plan…and he finally gave up waiting on me and walked it over himself in *April*. At least I rode my bike with him, so he wasn't alone.)

If you haven't heard of *The Five Love Languages*, I highly recommend it. Gary Chapman has variations for adults, singles, and kids. Knowing your love language might be helpful if you take on life changes like deciding to not buy anything new all year. For someone with a Words of Affirmation language, this presents the perfect time to share your love through homemade notes. If your love language is Physical Touch, well you can hug your gifts into each holiday.

For me, however, this was a challenge.

Not that gifts have to be new…but aren't they? I imagined myself handing a *previously owned* item to a friend on her birthday, sheepishly ducking my head into my hoodie and mumbling something about one man's junk and treasures galore, hoping she would open all of her gifts *after* the guests left to spare me public embarrassment. I mean, it's like giving *second-hand love.* Is there anything worse?

At the same time, I believed that this experiment creates space for creativity, for the support of local artisans, *and* to support what I'm sure were my friends' endeavors to reduce their own clutter. I certainly didn't want to be a contributor to their raised levels of stress by adding a new trinket to their shelf. How could I still show my love through my primary love language, yet honor our decision to buy nothing new? They seemed to collide in a conflict that would only end with my shame and embarrassment.

I decided to give everyone fair warning. Our kids. Our families. Our friends. I flew off a quick post on our blog about expectations. They could expect something not new. Somehow airing this out ahead of time made me feel less claustrophobic about our decision. Loved ones would now have the chance to squirrel my gift away and save me the public disgrace.

But that wasn't all.

We were also asking them to give *us* used gifts. Including our kids. Can you imagine telling grandparents to give their grandkids second-hand stuff for a birthday? If yours are already doing that, *rock on.* But I already mentioned my mom. Clearly my love language was genetic. Would people honor our request? What if they didn't? How would we respond? Would we let our kids keep the things? I really wasn't prepared for the idea of holidays and traditions within our experiment. It suddenly felt like we were destroying every friendship. Well, to me. My husband was thrilled.

I was also worried about traditions. Sure, a number of our traditions involve things we already own. Our advent book of mini Christmas books, classic stories of Christmas to read each day of the month, leading up to the biggest book, the Nativity story. Actually, we got this book from a thrift store…But I had other traditions. For example, from the time I was in high school, I'd made it a tradition to buy a stuffed animal *every time* I went to Disneyland. Okay, that wasn't *that* often, but it was something I did to mark my trip with friends or family. Or what about our Easter tradition of baskets with a new stuffed toy? Or stockings overflowing with end-aisle deals? What about *my* birthday and the tradition of giving me gifts? (Come on, before you think me too materialistic, I get three days a year to be celebrated *with* my love language in mind. I savor the feeling that people were thinking of me (more than the actual gift itself)).

Well, we'd take each holiday and each tradition as it came. And we'd be creative. For example, early on we decided that our only exception to "new" would be something handmade by a local artist. It's not mass-produced, and it supports the livelihood of someone. That's all win in our books.

We could also create from what we already had. We would dig deep into our wells of creativity and delight even ourselves at what had been buried beneath quick access to Walmart and Target. I already knew that my husband was creative, but the things he *made* from sticks in our yard or metal in our garage or old, discarded pieces of *who-knows-what* became these incredible, personalized, unique opportunities to show our care for someone. Instead of hiding my head in shame over gifts we gave, I held my head proud at the care our gifts took to find, create, and give.

We also discovered *causes*. Actually, that's what I did for one of my birthdays. I asked friends to donate to a cause of my choice (That year I chose HaitiGo, which I'd mentioned earlier) and they did. And in fact, more friends donated than who normally give me gifts. And you know what? I felt an abundance of love. It's not the *thing* that makes me feel loved. It's that someone was thinking of me and acted on that thought. And the number of people who supported my cause *also*, surprising to me, supported my need to feel loved through gifts.

Where I started out really nervous about how a year like this would go for a Gift-Giver like me, I ended the year blown away by the imagination of our family. I would never have seen what we could do together if we'd just kept on with our usual habit of running to the store or Amazon to buy the top item on the wish list. In many ways, I had a chance to demonstrate my love and affection for friends and family even *more* by spending thoughtful time on each gift. Some of those gifts came brand new from the thrift store. You would not believe how many sealed and wrapped items are being sold second-hand. Talk about national excess... we give away what we have before we even use it! Some of those gifts came from a local artist. And some of those gifts came from artists within my own home. Everything we gave had meaning and intentionality. And everything we received was the same.

It was way easier than I expected to find previously owned gifts that could be repurposed. My blog posts detail the things we found for various holidays. I remember leaving my favorite thrift store, Neighborhood Thrift, with bags full of Christmas gifts that my kids wouldn't even know were used. Or, even better than whether it still sparkled or smelled like cellophane were the gifts that looked used but were exactly the thing they would love. I was appalled at how much you can find in second-hand stores, including still-in-bag Easter grass and baskets. For reals.

The other things that shocked me was how on board our kids were. They were still pretty young at the time, one, three, ten, and eleven. But they didn't balk even once at receiving second-hand or hand-crafted gifts that year. Or in the years after (yep, the habit followed us). And they began to delight in finding the perfect treasure that might bless someone. This was a huge gift to me in and of itself: that my kids would continue to know they were loved *and* "buy" into our crazy idea and make it their own. I think some of their most memorable and favorite gifts came from this year.

I was also surprised at how much this ended up inspiring our friends and family. Sure, some of them struggled to know what to get our kids for birthday parties, but for the most part, people were more than happy to find a no-longer used toy in their home and pass it on. It became a gift to them to save money *and* get rid of something, and simultaneously see another child enjoy it. This was *really* evident at my annual Stay-at-Home Mom's Work Party during Christmas. (Yes, I was upset we didn't get work parties like Go-To-A-Job parents, so I created our own party). Typically, in the previous years, we all brought a new gift and had an exchange with the kiddos. But this year, I had to figure out how to orchestrate this while honoring our commitment. Fortunately, all the moms were on board. We all found nice but no-longer-played-with toys in our own homes, wrapped them up, and brought them to the exchange. It was *amazing* to see how each kid ended up with exactly what they would have wanted had they chosen! Each child's discarded toy became someone else's favorite toy. It was so meaningful (and who doesn't like both saving money *and* exchanging toys versus adding to the collection) that we continued in following years just like this.

Finally, I think I was surprised at how much God seemed to care about my little ol' feelings. He could have been like, "Marcy, gifts are so vain and selfish. It's about time you learn a new love language anyway. Pull up your panties and start serving." Strangely, that sounds more like *my* internal voice than the voice of God. But sometimes I mix them up. But then we have Christmas parties like that one, where each kid, regardless of gender or age, picked the toy from the pile that delighted them, and I can't help but think, *God? Is that You? Do you care for these kids and their silly little gift exchange?* Or the time we made photo valentines (Oh my word, they were so cute) and shared them with friends and family. *God? Do you really care about valentine's cards?* Or the time I really wanted an immersion blender, but didn't need it, and resolved to live with not ever finding a used one. And then the crazy story of one showing up. *God? Do you really care about my little wants that aren't even needs? Do you see and provide for those too?*

Friends, I'm here to say *yes*. If nothing else, this year taught me how much He sees and cares for every little thing.

So, we made it through the holidays, six of our own birthdays, and numerous traditions. But could we make it through *traveling*? We *love* to travel and wanted to move away from giving physical gifts to giving experiential gifts. Gifts that would last in our memories and photos as time spent together, living life together, delighting in each other. But how do you travel as a family and not buy new things? What about my Disneyland toy?! The next chapter will show you how we navigated being an adventurous family even while being a non-consuming family!

Blog Post—December—Used Gift Exchange

I miss work parties. Of all the things I love about getting to stay home with my kids...that one thing is true. I miss work parties.

So last year I decided to start an annual "work" party for stay-at-home moms. Apparently, it was a hit, because I was getting emails in early December about plans for this year's party!

Well, we had it. And it was fun.

Ten mommies. Twenty-three children. It was awesome.

One of the fun things we do at this party (other than eat and chat) is a used gift exchange for the kids. We each find a toy at home that isn't played with anymore. We wrap it up (one per child) and give it away. It's great. Many of the kids even get in on the "give-it-away" part in anticipation of the "new" toy they will receive.

We throw all the gifts into the middle of the room (that's twenty-three, mind you). Then we say "Go!" Sounds like chaos, right? It is. Fun, crazy, loud, sensational chaos. And that's just the moms!

Actually, it goes fairly well. The younger kids need a little prodding, but in the end, each child has a gift of some kind. This year was especially touching to me.

I had a brand-new Pluto plush that had been sitting in a bin. I actually have about three Plutos so decided this one could go. Since it still had its Disney tag, I tried selling it. No luck. Thank God! I threw it into a gift bag and gave it away. The sweet little boy who just *happened* to pick that bag was *thrilled*! It so happens that his favorite character is Pluto! I couldn't have asked for a better home! I never would have known to give it to him otherwise—what a joy!

My little Hannah picked a bag that had a mini Toys R Us inside. Books, dolls, clothes, mechanical toys. (That family cleaned out well!) I pulled out a couple of things for Hannah and then let the other twenty-two kids pick what they wanted. It was so cute. The same little boy with the Pluto kept asking, "I can have *two* things?" Another little girl pulled a Strawberry Shortcake doll from Hannah's bag. Little did I know that Strawberry Shortcake was her favorite character as well!

Finally, Corban, my three-year-old, was among the last to pick a gift. Someone found one left labeled "Toddler boy." It was between that one and the one *we* had brought, so he took that one.

Well, it happened to be a never used (it seemed) Disney *Cars* book...complete with a whole set of mini cars and a floor map to play on. If you know my son, you know that this was *his* gift.

I sat back at the end of the party and was filled with such joy. One person's "junk" was another person's newfound cherished treasure. What delight! And, not to sound cliché, but I was so blessed by how God had so lovingly arranged the gift of each child. True, some kids were initially disappointed...maybe they got a baby toy and they were quite a bit older than that. Still, they all left with something special—whether it was traded, given, or found.

The smiles were mesmerizing, and I found my own self smiling all throughout the day as I thought about the various ways children had been blessed. Isn't God good?

And all from something used.

Blog Post—May—Resoluting in Disneyland

Yeah, you are reading that right. We went to Disneyland and worked *very* hard at not buying anything new. As a matter of fact, we worked hard at spending little to no money, period. Here is what we did.

First of all, we jumped on an opportunity that Disneyland offered: Give a Day, Get a Day. I think it's over now, but basically, they gave one million people the opportunity to volunteer for an approved day of service and in return, they gave a free ticket to the park! Jeremy and I and our two oldest children were so excited to help *friends* with a fundraiser for their domestic adoption. We made greeting cards for two hours and got tickets! (Just a note: we would have helped them regardless. The fact that Disney supported them was such a gift!)

We were able to get *all six* of us into the park *free*. Do you know how much money that saved? Almost $300. Amazing. Liz had never been to Disneyland (Hannah either) so it was especially neat to take them.

We paid for gas with a Visa Rebate I had received for $90. Money already spent that we used to fuel our vehicle. I made lunch and dinner for the road. We stayed with a dear friend in Costa Mesa, so our housing was free (along with a breakfast the next morning!). We slept and then headed to the park on Mother's Day. We paid $14 for parking. Then as we entered the park, we were each given a number of buttons—Celebration buttons (for Mother's Day), Volunteer buttons (for earning our tickets), and my other two got First Visit buttons for being newbies. Then, they gave mothers a carnation for Mother's Day! Those were all of our free souvenirs (not to mention the plethora of pictures we took!)

We bought *one* meal in the park, which totaled about $50 (ridiculous, I know) but used our saved-up yard sale money from a couple months back. Then we bought sandwiches as we drove home that night.

Sounds easy, maybe. But really—I have had a tradition my *whole life long* of buying a stuffed animal (big or small) with every visit to Disneyland. I didn't! And I'm okay with that. I grew up in San Diego so you can imagine how many of these "traditions" I've collected over the years. The kids were content with their autograph books that I had made for them, filled with signatures to pair with the photos we took. Our great friend Allison made all of the kids tie-dyed Disney-themed shirts. And the handmade autograph books cost $5 to make as opposed to the $10-15 for the ones at the park.

It was such a fun day and so inexpensive! I felt really good about our decision to stick to the "buy nothing new" plan. I think, in the end, we didn't have to use any of our month's income on the trip because we used my rebate card and our yard sale money, with some to spare! It's possible!

Blog Post—December—A Second-Hand Christmas

Well, I promised a post on how we did Christmas on a buy-nothing-new budget. Here it is!

To start, my love language is Gift-Giving. I best express my love for others by giving them little tokens of thoughtfulness, usually items that *click* when I see them, because of some personal joke, funny story, or it's *just them*. Not any gift will do. It can also be a card or a note—something that says, "I was thinking of you while we were apart." Equally, I *receive* love on this same level. My poor hubby.

Anyway, our resolution really put a good challenge on my gift-giving heart. The many thrift stores in our area and the craftiness of my husband made for an amazing second-hand Christmas.

We had decided in the past that we would give our children three gifts each: something they need, something they want, and a surprise. We want to love them with "things" but not overdo it. We also don't want to lose sight of the true purpose of Christmas—the *giving*. The Gift. So off I went to find gifts for my kiddos. Here's what we got.

For my one-year-old daughter: Amazingly enough, I found my little darling a baby doll cradle *new in its box* at Neighborhood Thrift. Hello? It had never been opened! At this very moment, around ten baby dolls are sleeping in it...at once. Very communal.

We also got her a little stuffed horse (compliments of her three-year-old brother) and a nutcracker from Target. I had searched nearly every Thrift store I could find for nutcrackers and couldn't find a single one! Apparently, people keep these. We went as a family and saw the Nutcracker Ballet this year, so I really wanted some token to remind them of that experience. It was only two dollars and they each got one.

My three-year-old son got some clothes (hand me downs from friends) which happened to have some of his most favorite characters: Disney's *Cars* and a dinosaur. He was thrilled. He also got a moose stuffed animal from a thrift store (that he had picked out), a kid's toolbox (from my MOPS group), and his own nutcracker. He seemed to be the most excited of all my children for his nutcracker. In fact, it followed him around for a bit.

My ten-year-old daughter got a nutcracker, a *bunch* of clothes (all from thrift stores, but many with new tags still on them). She was ecstatic. She also got a *Book of Classics for Girls* from Usborne Books and More. I bought this new at a home party. She offered a fund-raiser party (which I hosted) to raise support for my dear friends, the Gilmores, who are moving to Haiti. So even though I bought it new, it was to help raise money for friends, from a woman running an Usborne home-business. Can't pass up a chance like that! My daughter also got a tea set, *new in its box*, from the same thrift store mentioned above. She had attended a tea party birthday party this year and loved it. Finding this tea set was perfect!

My eleven-year-old son also got a nutcracker, a *Book of Classics for Boys* (from the same fundraiser), a ton of clothes, and a Yoda, *new in its box* from a thrift store. It was amazing how many *new* things I found at thrift stores! My kids could hardly tell their gifts were "used!"

For other family members, my husband made really cool bird houses from an old fence lying in our back yard. They were awesome. And I don't think I took a single picture. We also gave some cool goodie bags filled with ingredients to make certain meals, for example, a bag with all of the dry ingredients for chocolate chip cookies, or a soup, or hot chocolate, or cornbread, with a recipe. It's like a meal or snack in a bag. They were super fun to make and even more fun to give away!

So, it's possible. Aside from the $2 nutcrackers from Target, everything was "used." The best part was that my kids were thrilled. They loved their gifts!

Blog Post—January 2010—Haiti and Me

This project of living on used things seems more appropriate in light of the situation in Haiti. For those of you who don't know, my husband and I were down there in July with one of three mission teams sent by our church. The three teams combined helped build an orphanage, ran a music and fine arts camp, sports camp, Vacation Bible School, and spent time with the orphans who were to be living in the orphanage. Our church, the previous February, raised money for the orphanage, a church, sugar cane equipment, wells, and more. And now this terrible earthquake.

We've heard, so far, that our friends and all of the orphans are accounted for. Fortunately, the orphanage is in a town called Pignon some eighty miles north of Port au Prince. Still, dear friends of ours were in the capital for a number of reasons, one of which was to pick up a shipment of shoes (over 600) that our church gathered and sent.

When my husband and I left Haiti with our two youngest children, we left behind all of our clothes and shoes but one pair (what we had on). I was totally blessed to see a little boy in pictures wearing my two-year-old's clothing after we left. The earthquake and resulting devastation has weighed heavily on our hearts, as well as on the hearts of our teammates and church body.

I sit at home, glued to the news and Facebook, waiting for updates on friends or their family, crying over the pictures. The hotel I stayed in, the Karibe, is gone. That's so hard to fathom. It seems easy and awkward to walk away from the computer and pretend this horror isn't occurring in Haiti. Obviously, it never really leaves my mind, but how strange it is to gaze in shock at the destruction, and then pause to feed my children a meal so readily, or use the restroom with running water, or *know* that my family is safe and well wherever they happen to be, then to return to the computer and rejoin the world of Haiti through photos and friends. It doesn't seem fair—especially when I think of all of the people who can't just turn it off. They are *there* and stuck—with nothing.

I know this is heavy so far, but it's a heavy situation. Hopefully the load lifts a little here. Though I have everything and they have nothing in material terms, so many are finding relief in communing with one another and singing and wailing before the Lord. This is baffling our nation—how people who already had little and have lost what they had, including their family, shacks of homes, friends, are praising Jesus in the midst.

My dear friend Dorina reminded me of a powerful verse for this time. Isaiah 54:10 says, "'Though the mountains be shaken and the hills be removed, yet My unfailing love for you will not be shaken nor My covenant of peace be removed,' says the Lord, who has compassion on you."

God LOVES Haiti and His creations. And though we can't ever fully understand why He allows such calamities to happen, we *know* that He is good and His ways are higher than ours. We live in a fallen sinful world, yet we can praise Him still.

My point, as I process this in front of you all, is not why God lets bad things happen (though I will have my fair share of questions when I get to Heaven too).

My point is this: Even in a nation with such excess, we still have nothing if we don't have Jesus. I can have everything and have nothing. I can have nothing and have everything. I've had dear friends in Israel, Paraguay, Guatemala—from all over—envy my life as an American. A life with "freedoms" and the "American Dream." And monetarily, religiously, materially, there is truth to these privileges of America.

However, I have often envied *them*. The community they live in and rely on, their very deep relationships with one another, the way they *must* rely daily on the provisions of the Lord, the way they see His miracles, grand ones, in ways we've only hoped to, so much so that some of us even think God doesn't do miracles anymore.

Even in our excess we can have nothing. My prayer is that I may be like the Haitians singing in their perfect harmony, praising God in the storm, in the midst of questions, confusion, and chaos, in the midst of grief deeper than a heart can bear on its own strength—that I can yet praise Him.

Lord, may that be the story of my life as well. May I be like the Haitians, whom You love deeply and with compassion and mercy, when all this life has to offer is removed from me, that I will be found in Your presence—in the midst of rubble, dust, destruction—praising You.

Chapter 12

Travel

Travel. The word alone incites flutters of joy in my heart. Traveling with people I love? Even better. I couldn't imagine putting day trips or weekend trips on hold during our year-of-nothing-new. And in fact, I was awakened to the idea of using *experiences* as a gift instead of *things*. With a million ways to capture photo-memories, one can hold on to the joy of an experience long after it's lapsed. In fact, brain studies have shown that photos can illicit some of the same emotional responses as though you were back *in* the moment you captured.[1] Photos can be the gift that keep on giving.

Photos can also be the gift that *takes*. Studies have also shown a new phenomenon of people living behind the lens, capturing what's in front of them but not really experiencing the present moment. There's even a name for this because it's that legit. And I've experienced it. The Photo-Taking Impairment Effect is the result of your brain offloading responsibility for memory onto your camera, thereby making the details of the memory harder to recall.[2] There's definitely a beautiful balance between capturing a treasured memory and losing yourself in the possibility of a memory, never actually living *in it* or *through it.*

A variety of trip opportunities came up during this year. And because our bank account was doing better, we could afford to take some mini vacays, along with a bag of creativity. My heart loves a good adventure. The first opportunity came when my baby sister decided she was ready to see the Big Apple. I had been a time or two for writing conferences and really enjoy a good visit to New York City. So, I was more than happy to offer my services as her tour guide and travel-mate. From the start, I didn't imagine it being too difficult to *not buy* anything on my trip. While I love a good souvenir, I also hate spending money and needing more things to dust (though I might have one shelf that would argue with me).

What I was again confronted with is *impulsivity*. Ugh. There's all sorts of good psychology around why we give in to impulse shopping, much of which, again, the marketers are well aware of. From where a product is placed in the store, to your accessibility to *touching* it, to the price-slashed tag, to your anticipated mood while shopping, brands employ all their guns when it comes to getting your attention and the contents of your wallet. And it often works. Did you know that touching an item enhances your chances of buying it? That's why Apple loves to let you touch *everything* in their store. Studies show that touching an item creates an attachment between you and that thing.[3] Perhaps that's why every wise parent says, "Don't touch!" to their kids entering a store. We *thought* it was about not wanting to pay for something they break. But no, it was also to inhibit their already strong desire to nag us into an if-you'll-stop-asking-I'll-buy-it purchase.

New York City vendors are masters in disguise of the impulse-buy strategy. The "Seven Shirts for $10" sign beckoned me. I didn't even know I wanted seven shirts for $10 until the sign told me it was possible. Or the "Buy 5 get 5 Free" Statue of Liberty keychains, complete with light up torch. Who doesn't need *ten* Statue of Liberty keychains? My Gift-Giving heart soared to think of all the people I could *bless* with my thoughtful gift from NYC. I passed the aprons that would give me a Statue of Liberty body while I cooked. I looked down at my ticket to Ellis Island. I sighed. The pretty paper ticket with the ship image would have to do for my souvenir, tucked away for a photo album I'd probably never make anyway. I said a quiet goodbye to the taxi snow globe and made my way to the ferry. My sister reminded me that our social experiment was *good* and that if we needed to, we could find loopholes in the plan. Oooh, a thrift store, maybe? I could probably get seven "I heart NYC" shirts, though not for the $10 deal. We decided to keep our eyes out for second-hand stores. (By the way, it appears that New York City has very few, if any, second-hand stores).

Little did I know how that ferry trip to Ellis Island would remove any reminder of shiny trinkets that had only moments before held my attention. Walking the halls where so many asylum seekers and better-life-makers had held hope for a new dream was sobering. Not only because it's places like this one that have made America what she is—home to the stranger, but because one of those strangers was *ours*.

Raffaello Guiseppe Battolla had walked these very halls. Twice. Having boarded the Vincenzo Florio in Genoa, Italy on October 25, 1904, our

20-year-old great-great grandfather left his motherland for the ideals of free America. He stepped onto the same dock we'd just stepped on, and made his way with his head high, pushing back fear and breathing in hope that this would be the start of a new life. He'd left everyone behind. And other than one trip back as a 28-year-old married man, he'd never return to his homeland. He graced the halls of Ellis Island for a second time, via the Princess Irene, on May 18, 1912.

My sister and I poured over the logs of Ellis Island guests. Twelve million people had passed through this immigration station, 98% of them being allowed entry after quarantine, interviews, medical exams, and other rigors of entry.[4] There he was. There, in old ink, was the reality of our own heritage penned onto the lines of history. I looked down the long hall and imagined the line of weary travelers. Some would be denied entry. Where would I be had he been denied entry? Had his health been too poor, or his pockets too empty, how would our family story have unfolded differently? This moment, his experience in this facility, was pivotal for my existence. My sister and I looked at each other in silence. The unexpected power of this excursion was overwhelming. The flashy kitsch that had so enamored me an hour before had long lost its importance. The greatest souvenir I'd take from this place was having stood in my great-great-grandfather's steps and realizing what gratitude I owed him and this welcoming nation of the United States.

Years later I would have the chance to visit the docks in Genoa, where young Raffaello boarded The Vincenzo Florio and later, the Princess Irene. I'd travel to his hometown to see what he'd been raised to see. Why had he left? The wars would later tear through his village on the coast of Tuscany, but he would fight with the Americans. On the evening of our last day, my phone rang. Our Airbnb hostess said, "Marcy, I think I know your family. May I give them your number?" Moments later, a cousin I'd never met greeted me on the other end of my phone line. "Come, meet with us," he invited. You see, he was visiting his parents and homeland, now an immigrant to the U.S. himself. We hopped in the car for what would be a moment of all moments. They told the story of a long-lost relative who, generations before, had boarded a ship for America. He'd written for a while but as time passed, the communication diminished, ended. This cousin, when a young man and ready to see the world, was encouraged to go to California where the last letters from this long-lost ancestor had arrived. *I* was the missing piece of their puzzle. The descendent of their beloved son, brother, and cousin who'd boarded a ship and made a new life. How ironic that we'd all meet together in this tiny little village, and not in California. It seems we'd made our way home after all.

Moments like that outweighs *any* thing you could ever give me. No trinket could ever give me what those moments gave me. Marketers might understand impulse buys and how to capture my attention, but they'll never be able to capture my heart.

This came to the test once again on a family trip to Disneyland in California.

As I'd mentioned previously, I'd had a tradition of purchasing a new stuffed animal on every visit to The Best Place on Earth, no matter my age. The invitation to join family friends on this trip elicited excitement, and low-level panic. It's *hard* for me to loosen my hold on traditions, dumb as they might be. Maybe this comes from having moved around a lot as a kid…the scenery might change but the tradition, that I could take with me. I can't but hear the song *Tradition* from "Fiddler on the Roof." Of course, I've laughed with the best of them at this scene in the musical. But on the inside, I'm also caving in…yes! Traditions have kept me balanced!

That beings said, I was either going to adjust my tradition and exchange it for something better or something temporary or fail our experiment. I'm not a quitter, so I committed to giving it up. *Cue the tears of sentiment* Fortunately, we chose to share this experience with one of the most creative people I know, Allison. If I could have half of what she has in ingenuity, this would have been the easiest year of my life, and I'd be a highly productive and sought-after person. She's incredible. You can read the blog post for the details of that day (Blog Post—May—Resoluting in Disneyland!), but the highlight is this: we spent a total of $69 for all six of us to enjoy the day in Disneyland. That's the gas to get there, food, entry, and parking. That's the souvenirs (that we made), the buttons they gave us, the limitless fun we shared together. Okay, you can add a few dollars for the picnic meals I packed. And the majority of that money came from our yard sale profits from *getting rid of stuff*.

If you haven't heard of *The Happiness Dare: Pursuing Your Heart's Deepest, Holiest, and Most Vulnerable Desire* by Jennifer Dukes Lee, I highly recommend it. There's a free quiz you can take to learn your happiness style. "Happiness," the word, gets a bum rap. It's like the black sheep of the Joy family. It's dismissed as superficial, frivolous, and elusive. Yet, according to Jennifer, we all have regular experiences with happiness that are worthy of our time and investment. Not at the expense of joy, sure, it's important to be content regardless of circumstances. But sometimes it's okay to be just plain ol' happy. This book revealed that my happiness style is both *relating* and *experiencing*. Put the two together—a new adventure or experience with someone I love—and you might as well have given me a shot of crack. Or whatever you do with crack to feel good. Scrap the crack! Learn your happiness style and *invest in it*. I'm sure the high is way better, longer lasting, and less detrimental for your brain cells.

That day at Disneyland, watching us spend nearly nothing in dollars but spend everything in quality time together and with friends was a 100/10 on my happiness scale. That's pretty high. Now, your happiness may come in different forms. It might come in doing purposeful activity and accomplishing things. Yeah! Your happiness might be highest when you're creating happiness for others through helping, sharing, or serving. Or you might feel fulfilled just sitting around *thinking*, pondering the world and coming to conclusions. Or, like me, you might find great delight in experiencing new things or in doing life with others. Knowing what brings you happiness can help you question the messages you might hear from commercials and ads. Is that new product *really* going to make me happy? I'll tell you this, "buying stuff" is not on the Happiness Dare list of happiness styles. Just saying.

Rethinking how we travel and what we buy on trips was a huge gift to me during this year. I survived not buying a stuffed animal at Disneyland. And you know what? I haven't bought one on any trip since (which has been, like, four times). And my home, to be honest, is better for it. In fact, all those original stuffed toys I collected with my visits are now in new loving homes. At least that's how I like to picture them. Versus in the bottom of a landfill. I digress.

Each of my treasured toys is now someone else's treasured toy. They didn't need a new one, and neither do I. If nothing else has taught me this lesson, it's watching our fellow humans in other countries navigate their lack of material opportunity and their great joy anyway. During this buy-nothing-new year, a devastating earthquake hit Haiti, a place near and dear to our hearts and ministry. In fact, when you read the blog post (Blog Post—January 2010—Haiti and Me), you saw just how connected we were. Yet what brought me to tears wasn't the devastation (okay, that did have me in tears, too). It was the people dancing in the streets, singing with tears streaming down their face, songs of joy and praise to God.

What. In. The. World.

I'm a follower of this God to whom they sang, and I'd like to think that in some incredibly horrific tragedy, I'd take to the streets and sing. But aside from a mighty dose of the Holy Spirit filling me up with supernatural presence to pull me out of my self-made puddle of despair, I doubt I'd be praising God *first*. I'd get there, but not first. Not like the Haitians. Oh, they felt their grief. They weren't *happy*. This was not their Happiness Dare moment. This was the sudden and inexplicable loss of people they loved. Of fragile homes that had sheltered them. Of roads they'd walked. Of the animals or gardens that had fed them. The loss was indescribable.

And one thing I've observed is that sometimes, having less means that when it's taken away, you can sing. You can sing because it wasn't your value or your identity. *You* are still intact. The you that is worthy of all love and affection is untouched. In pain, yes, but no less *whole*. These Haitians sang to *my* soul, a song of true wealth. Something I sometimes lack, even as I'm surrounded by affluence and privilege.

I remember sitting with friends-like-family in Paraguay, the least developed nation of South America. My friends, if they *had* an income, made up to $3 a day. Unemployment in Paraguay ranges from 7-9%, higher in the barrios where I lived. Their creativity flourished, bagging water and freezing it to sell as ice. Getting second-hand clothing from nearby Brazil to sell to neighbors. Growing remedies for common and uncommon diseases. My friend-like-a-sister healed my wart with a leaf. There's a lot of "free" time in the barrios of Paraguay. So, we'd gather in rickety chairs in the yards of neighbors, and we'd pass the Tereré, a herbal drink like Mate, but using ice water instead of hot. We'd pass the same cup, the same straw, from mouth to mouth in a kind of foreign-to-Americans togetherness. I remember Oscar imagining what my life in America might be like, with big houses, and paved roads, and food you didn't have to kill yourself. Money to pay for electricity and water that flows all day long. His wistful look made me both smile and feel sad.

"Oscar," I said. "We do have a lot of stuff. And your house would fit in one room in a typical American house. And there's a lot of money to go around. And you know where it all goes? To bills. And debt. And taxes. And fees. And you know what else? People are drowning in the wrong things. In material goods, hoping they'll feel happy, but they don't. Our suicide rate is high, our depression rate is high. People are sad and angry and rich." His eyes were wide as I shared. He'd seen a few of my pictures from home, a world unlike anything he'd ever personally seen. He'd imagined the big space and how many of his neighbors could fit in the yard for a celebratory barbecue. Or how maybe, in a house like mine, his brother's wife and ten children would be able to share four or five rooms instead of *two*. "But, Oscar, you are *rich*. Really rich. You have relationships and community. You have neighbors you can call on. You have togetherness and belonging. We just have stuff."

It was eye-opening for the both of us. Yes, we have a lot to learn from each other. I understand their envy of many of our American freedoms. We *do* have opportunity. Rights. Privilege. But I envy them, too. Their simplicity. Their connection to other humans. We have a lot to gain from one another. And I pray they never trade the gift they have in exchange for the "American Dream."

This is what I took away from fellow sojourners this year. That quality truly is better than quantity. It's cliché, now. A saying. But let it sink in. What does a *quality* life look like to you? Have you ever stayed in an Airbnb with all your stuff far away, silenced by time and actual distance, and thought, *I could live like this for a long time?* I miss the days when all I owned fit into a duffel bag.

The quality of our lives will never be measured in stuff. It will be measured in the quality of our human relationships. It will be measured in the foundation of our worth and value, which we simply *hold* without earning. It's measured in the song I sing when the world has crumbled around me. It took a global pandemic in 2020 to remind the *entire world* the power of togetherness. With shelter-in-place orders mandated in country after country, people *felt* the impact of social distancing and isolation. In countries like Paraguay or Italy or Kenya, where community is ingrained in daily life, the pandemic was emotionally catastrophic, perhaps even more than the virus that closed us all down to begin with. Even in countries where relationships are kept at arm's length, it felt emotionally claustrophobic. We remembered the power of *together*. And it mattered. And it made some of us not want to go back to the normal that had collided with the global shut down order. To rebuild with relationships at our core instead of the next shiny object, or level of achievement, or dollar bill.

It's your turn. You get to decide the quality of the life you'll live. Resist the impulse-purchase monsters biting at your neck to take your money in exchange for the life you want to live. Travel. Sing. *Belong* somewhere, to someone. This is what matters.

Now that I've left you with such a powerful call to action for your own life, I have to share with you where we failed. Has this been shiny so far? This story of successfully living according to our buy-used strategy, complete with all our successes, takeaways, and character development? Well, there were also missteps, fallaways, and character disappointments. And there was also grace, mercy, and learning. My friend Chandler Bolt of Self-Publishing School holds this as a company Core Value: Fail Fast, Fail Forward, Fail Often. Why? Because, he says, if we're not failing, we're not growing, learning, or improving the world around us. So, in the spirit of how failing is *forward*, I'll share with you all of our mistakes and what we did about it in the next chapter.

---

[1] Ewbank, M., Barnard, P., Croucher, C., Ramponi, C., & Calder, A. (2009, June). The amygdala response to images with impact. Retrieved May 22, 2020, from https://www.ncbi.nlm.nih.gov/pmc/articles/PMC2686226/

[2] Storm, B., & Soares, J. (2017, November). Forget In A Flash: A Further Investigation of the Photo-Taking-Impairment Effect. Retrieved May 22, 2020, from https://www.researchgate.net/publication/320994445_Forget_in_a_Flash_A_Further_Investigation_of_the_Photo-Taking-Impairment_Effect

[3] Perry, P. (2019, February 04). What we touch while shopping affects what we buy, researchers say. Retrieved May 22, 2020, from https://bigthink.com/philip-perry/what-we-touch-while-shopping-affects-what-we-buy-study-shows

[4] Kennedy, L. (2018, June 21). Most Immigrants Arriving at Ellis Island in 1907 Were Processed in a Few Hours. Retrieved May 22, 2020, from https://www.history.com/news/immigrants-ellis-island-short-processing-time

Blog Post—February—Love Cruise and Bahamas

The adoptions of our children were about to finalize in May. This was our way of celebrating their upcoming adoptions as a family.

Well, we did it! We were gone for eight days to Orlando, Florida and a cruise through the Bahamas. Again, I was faced with how easy it is to want to buy something *just because*. This was especially hard because I *love* music and was on a music cruise with some of my favorite artists in the world. I also really enjoy supporting them.

At the mention of supporting others, our family has discussed this alteration to our goal. We have decided that we can purchase items "new" if they are hand-made and support the livelihood of someone, something not mass produced. We ran this idea by our children on the trip. We try hard to not ever feel entitled to luxury. We *aren't* entitled (regardless of how one might feel). No one is. Not really. As we passed the impoverished homes of Bahamians and heard of their "need" to do and deal drugs to survive, peering into their shacks of homes, we found ourselves praying for these people. As we listened to the stories of the many staff on-board the ship, our hearts were broken with compassion. Jeremy was even able to share the gospel with his room attendant. The man had *never heard* the good news of Jesus and His gift presented before! And he was right under our noses.

My oldest daughter found a hand-woven purse that she liked. It had a Tinkerbell woven into it. As she checked it out and asked the price, I questioned the woman about her "job." She said that it takes two to three days to make a purse, depending on its size and design. The purse was only ten dollars. My daughter decided to purchase the purse and told the woman, "I am buying this from you for two reasons: One, I like it. Two, I know you worked really hard on it and I want to support you in your livelihood." The woman began to cry. So did my heart. THEY GET IT!

However, here is my confession. My husband's, really. I stayed onboard with the kids so they could nap (after a long tour of Nassau) and told him to go play. He left the ship and asked around about getting to a beach. After an ordeal, he made it to a beach—with no snorkeling gear. The snorkel tours wouldn't take him as a solo person and there was nothing to rent, only buy. So, he bought a snorkel. I wasn't thrilled when he told me he'd broken our family goal. But I realized quickly that messing up, changing things, and dissecting our family direction is all part of the experience. I hope that whoever he bought it from needed the money! And now we know to work out some possible scenarios in the future to be prepared for situations like his. He had spent *a lot* of time trying to get out there, that he finally figured to make it worth it, he'd just buy the thing and be on with it. All right! Onward we march!

Blog Post—January—New York-Fashion Capital of the World!

Hello again! I know it's been a couple of days. I went to New York City with my sister. I *made it*! I didn't buy a single thing. I hear the shopping deals are incredible. I wouldn't know. Some of you may be super impressed at the moment. "You went to NEW YORK CITY and didn't even walk into Bloomingdales? Macys? JC Penny? THE HERSHEY'S FACTORY?" As incredulous as that might seem—It's true. And also, I'm not a big shopper. The excessive stimuli gives me a headache.

The hard part for *me* was not buying a souvenir! My plan was to find a thrift store and then tell you how funny it was that I bought an "I LOVE NY" shirt from there—but nope. Plan fail. I only saw *one* thrift store the entire time I was there, and I was passing it on the tour bus. There were "cheap" gifts everywhere. I could get *seven* shirts for $10. Who doesn't need seven more shirts?

My tour guide assured us that we'd only get one wash out of those, but still. I *did*, however, take 400 pictures.

On that note, I again felt the weight of how easy it is to buy something *just* to buy it. I think, even though I didn't *need* anything (and I surely don't need another knickknack statue to remind me of a place), I *would have* bought something. A mini Lady Liberty. Some memento for the kids. The payoff was this: my family spent a good half hour together enjoying my photo slideshow and watching the videos (especially of our crazy cab ride!). That kind of gift to my family is worth far more than a re-made blanket of the *Titanic* or a jumbo souvenir mug.

That said, I'm glad I made it! My sister was good at trying to find ways to twist the rules, like: "I'll buy the $2 shirt, wear it, then sell it to you for a quarter!" Sweet girl. In the end, I realized New York had nothing that I *need*, but plenty to experience and enjoy.

More to come! OH, and I found a free used fireplace key! WHAT?! Amazing.

Chapter 13

That Time We Failed

The thing about perfectionists is that we, I mean, *they* strive for excellence and are highly motivated—and also burn out and deal with a lot of anxiety. Had I been a perfectionist (ahem), failing would have been out of the question. Failing would have meant *I am a failure.* It would have proved my deep, inner fear that I am somehow unworthy of love and affection. Failing equals being unlovable. Unlikeable. The scum of the earth. I mean, to perfectionists, that is.

Research shows that there are two kinds of perfectionism: excellence-seeking-perfectionism and failure-avoiding-perfectionism.[1] Ironically, the research shows that neither forms of perfectionism perform any better than those non-perfectionists. They simply bring high standards, excellence, motivation, and drive to their performance. And, they also bring workaholism and burnout from excessively high expectations of self and others.

You can imagine how, had I been a perfectionist, the idea of failing would have been detrimental to my view of self. Had I been a perfectionist, I would have set extremely high expectations for ourselves. I would have determined that we would *never* buy a new item, no matter the "cost" or benefit or circumstance. Because *what would people think of me?* What would *I* think of me?

Perfectionist or not, we all hear messages about our worth and value when we fail. It's the same reason we avoid pain. Failure feels like pain, so we avoid it. *Oh, you failed. That means you're a loser. All the evidence is right here—you're a fraud and you've been found out. Now you'll lose everything you love because #YouAreFailure.* Nope, no failing here.

Until February. That's right, we made it one whole month before our first failure. Yep, our *first* failure. And I should mention, for the record, that the failure wasn't directly mine (like the following two failures). It was my husband's. Had I been a perfectionist, I might have hated him for ruining our experiment one month into the journey. Hate is strong. Judged at a minimum.

You can read what happened in our blog post of that trip. It's unforgivable really. Until my personal failure.

At least *I* made it eight-ish months before my big fail. Remember my love language? Gift-Giving. Yep, it won. It won out over my commitment to our year of buying only used things. Even though eight months of gifts leading up had *not* won out over the commitment—this one did. My sweet almost-three-year-old was sick. The kind of sick you get when you overeat gummies at your big sister's birthday party when no one is watching. Gummies that had been swimming in cool whip while the guests were swimming in the pool. So. Many. Gummies. What my baby didn't know, that he now knows, is that those cute, chubby bear-faced gummies are only sweet going *in*. And a few too many equals Haribo's Revenge in all the worst ways. Cue my #mamaguilt for not watching him better during the birthday party. It was painful to watch him suffer, even if his toddler-size gluttony was the cause.

I was out of all the things that help tummies and guts (and the various ways those places expel their angry contents). I ran to the local store to get crackers and 7UP and whatever remedies my mom had passed down to me. And there it was—the shiny, prominent, end-aisle bin of discounted toys. (*Note—the marketers had to know some heartbroken guilty mom would be heading to the register and need a value-lift by purchasing their "discounted" item. Ugh. I'm a sucker.*) I saw Buzz and Woody. Two of my son's favorite characters from his then favorite movie, *Toy Story*. People, my son wore cowboy boots *everywhere he went*. Including with his swim shorts. He was in it for real.

Here they were. Staring at me. And I made a decision. I made the decision to fail our experiment to love my son. Sounds noble, right? I can spin it all sorts of ways to make it sound okay, but the reality is…he didn't need the toys. I could have loved him with my 7UP and crackers and hugs and he'd never have known different. Looking back, I was loving myself. Making myself feel better by assuaging the mama guilt *and* the helplessness I felt to make his agony end. That was it. I felt helpless. This was something I could *do*. Something I could give.

Now, had I been a perfectionist, I might have noble-ized my failure in order to make it not a failure. (Read the blog article.) But it was a failure. I succumbed to the marketing-schemes and my own deprivation. Was it the end of the world? No. No, the world kept turning, the manufacturers kept producing, and our experiment kept experimenting. Because the reality is, "Being brave means knowing that when you fail, you don't fail forever" (Lana Del Rey).

Overcoming failure is getting up, dusting yourself off, and trying again. It's learning your weaknesses and endeavoring to make them strengths. Failure is a catalyst for humility, one of the greatest powers in the world, and one so few have. I hate feeling humbled. It crushes in at all sides, threatening to expose me for the fraud I'm sure I am. Makes me *feel* the smallness and insignificance I run from every day. Many esteem humility as a sought-after character trait, yet run from its reality in their own lives. It's the hurts-good kind of pain. Except sometimes it only hurts.

If I were only left to the world's devices and definitions, humility would define me as finally knowing my low place in the world. Many esoterics would *pursue* humility as a sign of their lack of pride, their goodwill toward others, their self-sacrifice. This, in itself, can turn into pride. Yet in these moments of feeling humility weigh in on me, I'm reminded of a verse in the Bible, Proverbs 11:12, which says, "When pride comes, then comes disgrace, but with the humble is wisdom." Indeed, the "good" in the hurts-good pain of humility is the wisdom I gain. I learn something of myself when I fail, when I'm humbled. This learning becomes my strength, like a muscle that's been torn and repaired and grows now stronger. With this strength I step into my next obstacle, equipped with the humble lesson behind me. Will I be humbled again? Unfortunately-fortunately, yes. It's these humilities of the past that have, in mercy, brought me where I am today.

If anyone had been humbled, it was the brothers of Jesus, who though raised beside him with the stories passed down from their parents of His miraculous birth, still didn't believe (John 7:5) and called him "out of his mind" (Mark 3:21). Yet after the death of Jesus and His resurrection, all of the brothers come to belief in Him as the Son of God. Not only belief, but leaders and even *martyrs* for their belief. Talk about humility. James, one of his brothers, says, "But He gives more grace. Therefore, it says, 'God opposes the proud, but gives grace to the humble'" (James 4:6).

That is another gift of failing. Of humility. Grace. Grace and Mercy. Being both given what you don't deserve as a gift (forgiveness, maybe) and not being given what you *do* deserve (punishment). I know in the scheme of things, buying my son a new toy to ease his pain and mine isn't that big of a deal. But if I want the gifts that come with failing, I have to sit with it, small as it may seem. As Henry Ford is quoted as saying, "The only real mistake is the one from which we learn nothing."

My integrity was at stake. My honor was at stake. My commitments could be questioned. Or, so the messages in our heads tell us, right? That failure equals the loss of all we've worked so hard to build. Chris Hardwick says it one of my favorite ways, "No human ever became interesting by not failing. The more you fail and recover and improve, the better you are as a person. Ever meet someone who's always had everything work out for them with zero struggle? They usually have the depth of a puddle. Or they don't exist." As a writing coach, I often tell my student writers that relatability is credibility. That in our current world, we seem to care less about the letters after someone's name, and more about the real life they've lived. It turns out that our ability to rise from failure makes us the most relatable of all. I mean, who wants to listen to someone with the depth of a puddle?

Well, apparently failing twice wasn't enough humility. There was failure number three. And this failure was a good teacher. The longer version of the story is in the blog article, but the gist is this: busy mom, lots of kids, rushing, rain, cold, sweater-less toddler, no time to go home. *sigh* In order to not drop off my child for a half day of *no warmth* on a rainy day, I drove to Walmart. And for the low price of $6, was able to dress my kiddo and get him back to school. Honestly, I don't regret it. I learned that sometimes failing is the right thing to do. And sometimes there is grey area in our black-and-white experiments.

"Failure should be our teacher, not our undertaker. Failure is delay, not defeat. It is a temporary detour, not a dead end. Failure is something we can avoid only by saying nothing, doing nothing, and being nothing" (Denis Waitley). That day, in my detour from our family commitment to buying-used, I realized that sometimes I'm grateful for the mass-production of commercial items. Or, at least the fact that they open earlier than my second-hand options. It's easy to be do-or-die or all-or-nothing. But in reality, life has so many caveats.

When I think of grey areas in life, I want to throw in the rag. For example, putting an end to commercialism and mass-produced junk feels good to me. It feels healthy and whole and worthy of my attention. And then global pandemics show what happens to an economy, and thus to families, and then to whole nations, when our flow is disrupted. In the pandemic of 2020, businesses the governments deemed as "non-essential" were closed down. (Don't get me started on what was deemed essential or not.) Amazon drastically reduced the shelving of non-essential items and, if you could order it at all, delivery was deprioritized. In some ways, this could seem like an answer to the stop-consumerism prayer. But how it played out was with over 30 million people losing their jobs. Half of every household had someone lose their position or get a drastic pay cut.[2] This included my sister, who manages a gym. My dear friends who run their own Web design and video production company. This includes my mom, who works in a school kitchen. This includes my sweet friend, who is a hairstylist. My other friend, who owns a restaurant. The impact was much greater than just commercial items, but the reality was, I never would have *considered* the loss of jobs connected to my "shut-down-mass-production" movement.

It's easy for me to follow the rabbit trails of all we fight for, only to be overwhelmed by the nuances and caveats. It makes me want to quit and say, "I'll never know the right answer that ends global harm by not preventing *different* harm." In my fear of causing harm by ending harm, I quit. But "I'd rather be partly great than entirely useless" (Neal Shusterman). Does that mean we don't think conscientiously? No way! We still do our homework. But we don't fall into overwhelm and quit because of fear. In fact, a quote that hangs above my office desk is by Nelson Mandela. He said, "May your choices reflect your hopes, not your fears." This has become my mantra.

Choosing my hopes over my fears silences a lot of the argument. When I have to face my biggest critic (myself) and I intentionally choose *hope* over fear, suddenly my critic shrinks back defeated. The messages that shame my worth and value are *all* based on fear. Every one. But when I say, *No! I choose hope!* There's no power left. When I look the possibility (inevitability) of failing in the face, and choose hope, failing becomes a steppingstone. Johnny Cash said, "You build on failure. You use it as a steppingstone. Close the door on the past. You don't try to forget the mistakes, but you don't dwell on it. You don't let it have any of your energy, or any of your time, or any of your space."

When I choose hope, I can look at grief and loss, as many experienced in the pandemic, and know that it's not the end of the story. I can sit in the pain, feel the pain, and release the pain to the lesson it has for me, because hope tells me there's more *good* around the corner. I can, with hope, change my opinions or plans toward solutions that serve us all the best. I can realize that while commercialism is a beast (I still believe that) it provides a lot of jobs and incomes for families I love. Maybe, says hope, the answer isn't all or nothing, but a balance.

Fear would have me accuse and judge and condemn. But hope gives space for conversation. Hope takes us beneath the surface levels where fear has kept us chained, and asks the big question: Why? And we dig and we wrestle with the *why* until, muddy-faced and filthy, we remember why we started. And we remember the beauty of mercy and grace.

These failures taught me that "Success is not final, failure is not fatal: it is the courage to continue that counts" (Winston Churchill). And continue we did, beyond our failures, into a greater awareness of who we are and the novelty of the world around us.

Whatever failures led to the pandemic of 2020 also led to the revelation of much of humanity's beauty. Our ugliness, too, but fear always keeps our ugliness evident. It's beauty which often gets pushed down, suppressed. Sometimes in our internal or external pandemics, we get to rise up and shine. And shine so many did. Nurses and doctors who put the lives of others before their own. People in large cities around the world singing to and with each other from their balconies, forbidden from leaving or touching, but not from meeting in the sky. Neighbors offering to shop for the immunocompromised and elderly to protect them from germs at the store. Churches, forbidden from gathering, but joining in common purpose to *feed* entire communities during the hardship. Families trading in busyness for mandated togetherness, remembering the joy of belonging and a slower pace. So many people sewing masks to aid healthcare workers who didn't have any. On and on it goes. People choosing hope over fear. Moving forward with failure. "It's not how far you fall, but how high you bounce that counts" (Zig Ziglar).

And just as our own failure found us and taught us, so did many surprises and delights along the way. See, that's the other thing about not quitting, about choosing hope over fear. It makes room for the unexpected waves of beauty and connection that we otherwise would have missed. In the next chapter, I share the miracles and surprises that blew our socks off and often brought me to tears. Who knew what an adventure this year would hold for us?

[1] Swider, B., Harari, D., Breidenthal, A., & Steed, L. (2019, November 26). The Pros and Cons of Perfectionism, According to Research. Retrieved May 23, 2020, from https://hbr.org/2018/12/the-pros-and-cons-of-perfectionism-according-to-research

[2] Lacy, B. (2020, May 02). Business Report: 30 Million Americans Lose Jobs During COVID-19 Shutdown. Retrieved May 23, 2020, from https://www.kpbs.org/news/2020/may/01/business-report-30-million-americans-lose-jobs-dur/

Blog Post—October—Convenience Culture Pay Off

I was humbled on Tuesday.

Actually, I find some humility every day.

Tuesday was different.

I had to take my older kids to school (which is unusual for me, usually my hubby takes them). This meant getting my older two in the car and ready to go. I had to get my two babies in the car (wake them up and feed them). I had to get my son's preschool stuff together. Throw in my guitar and Bible study book for Bible Study at nine. Oh, and the juice I had to bring for potluck.

All that to say, by the time we got to my son's little preschool, it was raining. Add to that—of all the things I could have forgotten that morning, it happened to be his backpack, complete with sweater and umbrella. Yep. Fortunately, we were half an hour early. I quickly (but not too quickly) drove to Goodwill. CLOSED. Actually, just about everything was closed at 8 a.m. (Really? When did all of the businesses decide 9 a.m. and 10 a.m. were better times to avail themselves to frantic mommies of cold children?) The only place open: Walmart.

In we went! Six dollars later we had a great warm sweater. We made it back to his school just in time for his class to start. (A couple days later I found a light rain jacket at Neighborhood Thrift. Score!)

As you know, Walmart is *not* on our list of places to buy "used" things from. However, on this day, I was reminded that our culture of convenience isn't *all* bad. It sure comes in handy in those emergencies that don't leave you much time for bargain and thrift shopping. And I still got a great deal!

I love when God restores balance to my little universe. I needed to remember that every *new* purchase is not a bad purchase. Not every transaction of convenience is utterly detestable or ridiculous. It seems He certainly uses these methods to meet our needs as well as the others we are experimenting with this year! May the Lord lead and guide you as you wait on Him for your every need!

Blog Post—August—Birthdays, Birthdays, and More Birthdays.

Wow, it's been a while since my last post. Whoops!

Here's why: I've begun homeschooling my 11-year-old, which I believe will be short-lived. I have two toddlers. I've been invited to lead worship for my Bible Study which means I have to dust off the guitar and learn some songs. I'm a wife. I live in a house with five other people, a dog, and a cat (though the animals stay outside). I am a writer. I'm the publicity coordinator for my Mothers Of Pre Schoolers group. All of these are great blessings. All of these use up my resource of *time*.

That said, it's 11:02 p.m. The kids are asleep. The cat is asleep. The dog is asleep. The hubby is working on school stuff. My guitar is locked up. My MOPS work is done (for the time being) and I'm ignoring the unswept floor. Finally, my laptop is open before me. Here we go.

Since my last post we've had at least three more birthdays, a child with a tummy ache (too much candy at one of the parties), an entire summer, and the beginning of the school year. *Crazy!* I mention the tummy ache because it was the only time (in these last months) where I chose to break our resolution...for the love of a child.

Unfortunately for this resolution, my love language is gift-giving. My then 2-year-old had snuck a gummy bear too many and his body was working it back out...of both ends. Sorry for the details. We moved him to our room so he could wake us up if he needed to. Did I mention he was potty training? (side note: he woke up one day and agreed to "no more diapers" and now won't let us put one on him if we try! He made it through the above episode without *one* accident! He woke us up in time to make it to the potty!) Back to the confession. He needed some crackers and 7-Up...both of which I was out of. So, at 1 a.m. I headed to my neighborhood 24-hour Winco. God bless that store.

While there I saw a Buzz and Woody toy. I'd passed it a bunch of times knowing that I "couldn't" buy it out of loyalty for our decision. This time, however, I made the conscientious decision to love my baby boy with a new gift. Hearing him cry as his gummy bears punished his gut broke my heart and my resolution. I came home to a sweet son, dealing ever so gracefully with his situation, and gave him the *new* Buzz and Woody. He slept with them that night and recovered very well from his tummy trouble. It made me happy to see him happy in a moment of such discomfort and pain...it was worth the break from our goal.

Aside from that, though, we've really stuck with it! I've discovered some of the best thrift stores in town...and re-realized that I'm a yard sale junkie...so I'm not sure if this whole plan is helping my budget yet or not! We've had an Olympic-themed party, a Caribbean-themed party, and a Lion King party...all using previously owned or handmade items. Even the gifts were either used or food. I've bought some beautiful handmade tutus from a friend as gifts for other little girl toddlers. SO cute.

I stayed up till midnight making Pride Rock. Fortunately, I had the right Lion King toys already to complete the scene. My son loved his cake. He's three, so it didn't have to be amazing to anyone but him.

I also made dirt cupcakes! We all enjoyed some "grub" with Pumba and Timon. Favors were animal crackers in some safari-themed favor bags (last minute compliments of a friend, thanks!).

This has been the year of making fun cakes (and I am not a baker). My husband is "from" a Caribbean island, San Andres. This was an ode to his islander side. Everything was edible... palm trees were made up of biscotti, bubble gum leaves, and white chocolate glue. Coconuts were chocolate covered raisins. The sand was ground up animal crackers. And of course, gummy sharks and fish.

We had an Olympic-themed birthday party for my oldest daughter. So much fun! We made all of the medals and awards with chocolate coins. We are still continuing to learn so much in this process. I'm still blown away by how easy it is to go meet our own needs and rob God of the opportunity to do it. Not that He doesn't sometimes meet our needs through Target...but I've had some really neat experiences waiting on Him. And it's still amazing how much stuff we have. Every time we have a yard sale or give something away, I think: "Okay, now I *really* have given everything I don't want away." And then someone says they need something, I happen to have it...and it's gone. OR I just get in a mood of "that's gotta go." We will be having another yard sale in two weeks.

Thanks for patiently waiting for me. I'm not sure who I'm thanking really...maybe just the Internet abyss out there...but regardless, it's good practice.

Chapter 14

Takeaway

Not only was learning to fail (and the lessons we learned *from* failing) life-changing, but in many ways, the whole year's experience was life-changing. I'm sure our one year of intentional not-buying-new didn't make a noticeable impact on the national economy, but it made an impact on our own. Not just the economy of our wallets and bank accounts but on our hearts as well.

For one, we learned how tied we were to stuff, even though we would have said otherwise. We played with new, fun ways to spend our money, like causes we believe in or experiences together instead of toys that will break or lose the interest of their owner. My impulse to get in my car and drive to my local mass-production center was strong. Or if I felt super lazy or inept, I'd want the ease of a click on Amazon. It was my default response to recognizing I wanted or needed something. Even after some really cool experiences *because* of not giving into the impulse, I still found myself at times begrudging that I had to do this the *difficult* way. Or sometimes even the more expensive way. Items at Goodwill are sometimes more expensive than they are next door brand new. Yet as time passed, and I created a community of like-minded people on Facebook and found second-hand resources I loved, it became easier and more joy filled.

I was also surprised to find how guilt-free I felt providing for my family. Impulse buys often leave me with shopper's remorse. But having to spend so much time searching for an item gave me plenty of time to think about how much I actually needed it. Sometimes I realized I didn't, and that felt like a win in and of itself. Other times, when I found it, the story surrounding my discovery was such a high that I didn't regret the item itself.

Which leads to the blessing of the discovery. Time and again, the *journey* to the item was so rewarding. Yeah, there were bumps and hurdles, but for the most part, I felt so connected to other humans, my own family, my own need, and the *process*, something I rarely experience with my quick jaunt to Target. My blog articles on the journey to paper or to the immersion blender, are just examples. You better believe that my experience with those two items has forever changed how I see and experience them. Seriously, every time I use paper or blend up a delicious soup, I'm overwhelmed with gratitude. They're not even the originals anymore…I've moved on to "new" used immersion blenders and (store-bought) paper, but they consistently ensure a sense of gratitude in me. Remember how gratitude and worry can't co-exist in the same moment? The more that I let into my house that holds the power of gratitude and joy for me, the less I can stress about *anything*. I did not see that coming.

Living lives of entitlement, pride, and arrogance often prevents the gift of gratitude. So does living a life of worry, stress, and anxiety. Gratitude is the antidote to so many ailments, and who knew the gift of it was in the journey of acquiring what we own? Living lives of humility, failure, and wonder, often invite gratitude and wholeness. This doesn't mean we now need to create journeys of acquiring in order to experience a journey that leads to gratitude! You can cultivate gratitude with what's right in front of you. In the book, *One Thousand Gifts: A Dare to Live Fully Right Where You Are,* author Ann Voskamp talks about the power of slowing down and truly *seeing* what you have. She said, "The brave who focus on all things good and all things beautiful and all things true, even in the small, who give thanks for it and discover joy even in the here and now, they are the change agents who bring fullest light to all the world." Living gratefully makes us slow down and live *intentionally.* Fully alive and present. It's terrifying.

Slowing down and choosing gratitude for what *is* means making space for our fears and doubts and insecurities to access our minds. They shout louder as they clamor for our attention. Isn't that why we're so busy? To drown them out? Yet it's the bravery of stepping into the quiet of now that releases gratitude and joy. The choosing of *hope* over fear is the courage that fuels all joys that follow. Sometimes the joy and gratitude are on the other side of failure and pain, yes, and our fearlessness to take it on castrates the power they hold over us. This is something our experiment showed me. The power of slow (which I used to hate) and the power of gratitude (which used to elude me). They say comparison is a joy-killer. It's also a gratitude-killer. You can't be thankful for something you have if you're envying someone for what you don't have. There was no need to compete with the Joneses because our priorities were now different.

Priorities and personal values are the roots of a tree. When we look around our society, we see such polarities of strife and conflict, and selflessness and generosity. Why? What is the root motivation for how people choose to live out these few days we've been given? Researchers have determined that there are some foundational commonalities that motivate humans, like having *purpose*, and experiencing *mastery* and *autonomy*.[1] These may manifest differently depending on whether you're being driven by intrinsic or extrinsic motivation, your personality, your life experiences, your level of resilience, your fears, etc. But generally, we all want to survive, contribute to the world around us in some way, and experience love and connection. Sometimes, in our hunt for these things, we manifest anger and violence, and sometimes bravery and others-oriented living.

Our own motivations came under scrutiny during this year. This caught me by surprise. I thought of myself as a nice person, who loved to help others and had a high capacity for productivity. This year exposed me. On the surface level I was those things, but deeper down I was a slave to the messages around me about my beauty, my intrinsic worth, my lovability, and my contribution (or lack thereof) to the world around me. These messages were the masters of my puppet strings. Why did I buy what I didn't need? Collect what didn't satisfy? Spend more than I made? Because I was trying to prove my value and my status, to those around me, sure, but mostly to myself. During our experiment, I was refused access to my normal means of providing value to myself, and this was so, so good. It gave me time to slow down and see myself *truly*, without the lens of competing messages, and what I saw had so much potential. So much beauty.

This came in part by seeing how God met every need the whole year, down to the smallest details and heart desires. Would He lavish such love on someone without value or worth? He makes me beautiful. He gives me every ounce of worth I hold. Without Him, I really *am* nothing. Dust returning to dust. But He infuses His image into each of our hearts and we become His reflection. How can the messages of this world compete with that of a most high God and loving Father? It can't. As I slowed and paused and reflected, I could see His lavish love poured out all over me. I was powerless to orchestrate the details that came together as they did. I could only sit back and marvel at His care and attention to detail. Want to feel overwhelmed with gratitude? Even in a broken and confused world? Spend some time looking for His fingerprints on your life. It changes everything.

Though the impact of this year can hardly be noticed here, I can't skip over the impact on our kids. They didn't really have a choice. Even so, they embraced the year in ways I couldn't even have really asked them to. From our daughter's desire to bless local artisans in impoverished countries (where most people go for luxury and miss the actual *humans* on the fringe of their vacation), to their reception of repurposed gifts, to the "noes" they faced with every, "Can I get that?" at the store. They not only blossomed in their own creativity and gratitude, but they also witnessed God's love poured out on them as individuals. Who knew an experiment like this would so radically change the hearts of a family? Only the One who inspired the idea from the start.

In the next chapter, I'm going to let my kids tell you for themselves. We interviewed them at the conclusion of the year to hear their hearts on the experience: the good, the bad, and the ugly.

---

[1] Pink, D. H. (2009). Drive: The surprising truth about what motivates us.

Blog Post—October—Celebrating for a Cause (Other Than Myself)

Finally, of the gazillion birthdays we've celebrated this year, mine came around!

I love my birthday. Not just because I get to be the center of attention for a little while, but because I have a scheduled reason to spend time with friends! Lots of them, all at once! Or, I have some excuse to do something ridiculous in the name of my birthday. Last year, we went to Medieval Times all dressed up—that was great.

This year, however, was the big 3-0. My husband and a dear friend, Dorina (along with some faithful helpers), jumped onboard for throwing me a party. It was filled with delicious food and tons of fun games based on the "Minute to Win It" game show. I had never actually seen the show, but it was so much fun!

As far as gifts go, we've been trying to figure out how to handle gift-givers in light of our resolution. For a couple birthdays (maybe all of them?) we asked people to give previously loved gifts rather than buying anything new. We didn't want people to spend money on new things for us since we weren't doing it for ourselves. Besides, when their birthday comes around, they are getting something used (or handmade) from us!

Facebook Causes sent me an email about having people donate to a cause in lieu of gifts. What a great idea! So, I set up a birthday wish. I decided to try to raise $500 for my friends who are moving to Haiti. They have had long standing relationships and history (like, for generations) and now are wanting to go and *live* the need they keep hearing about from their dear Haitian friends. They have been to Haiti numerous times. In fact, my family joined them on a ten-day trip to Haiti during the summer of 2009. This has given us a heart-connection with the people as well.

But I thought, why stop there? I asked *all* of my friends to send gifts to my Birthday Wish instead of purchasing me a gift.

I must state here that my "love language" is gift giving. Not so much for the sake of the gift as much as for the knowledge that someone has been thinking of me. I laid that "love" aside for this Cause only to be completely taken by surprise. It has been *so* neat to see people respond!

I've received donations for my birthday from people who don't normally get me a gift. I think I feel *more* loved by the response to the Birthday Wish than I ever would have from the traditional gift-giving of birthdays!

Anyway, I've been so blessed by this experience that I've decided to support a cause for *every* birthday here on out. Not only that, but my husband has been inspired to do the same. It's so exciting to see people give in my "honor." I'm hoping and praying that my children see the joy that overflows from celebrating one's birthday in this way and will thus become creative about how to celebrate their own!

In conclusion, I've known a number of people to use their birthdays to raise money for causes or to help the less fortunate. Here's a shout-out to everyone who already does that! I GET IT!

Blog Post—November—Candy Buy-Back

We caught wind that a dentist (Dr. Treva) was giving children *money* to sell her their Halloween candy. What a brilliant idea! A candy buy-back! We, just like *most* parents, would love a good way to keep our children from eating all of that Halloween candy. Or maybe it's just me. As a child, I saved my Halloween candy all year. Not only was I a little savorer (enjoying special pieces only on occasion) but I lack a sweet tooth. My friends *loved* this about me. Every time they came to visit, I still had Halloween candy to share!

So maybe I'm just a nerd. But I jumped on this opportunity to sell all of their candy. In we went, a one-year-old, three-year-old, ten-year-old, and eleven-year-old, all bogged with bags of candy. Yes, even my one-year-old. Because she's so cute, candy distributors inundated her bag with sweets, regardless of her limited teeth to even chew it. I digress.

Dr. Treva bought their candy for $1 per bag. We made out of there with $5! Last year, we let the kids pick as many candies as they were years in age. Then we traded the rest for Jamba Juice. This year, we forgot about letting them pick out some and just sold it. Then we went to the Dollar Store (not a thrift store, but almost!). I let them each pick something with their dollar and offered to cover their tax. This way, each child had something tangible and fun. My oldest bought sunglasses. My next oldest bought fake money with a money tray (and kindly paid for the dinner I made her). My youngest son bought a paddle ball. And my baby couldn't decide, so she kept her buck. And because it's the Dollar Store, it's all only going to last a couple of days *anyway* and will then make it to the trash—minus the cavities, obesity, and sugar highs. (Point in case, the ball and the paddle parted ways after only four hours).

I just wanted to share another really cool way to have a "loose" hold on things in life, including our candy mountains. Maybe my "sweets" aren't actual sweets...maybe it's my laptop, or my iPod, or my guitar, or *whatever!* Maybe it's even my children! But to truly be at peace with our lives and the journey God takes us on, we have to hold things loosely, for the season with which we've been given them.

I loved seeing my kids so willing to give up all that candy for only a buck. Oh, and for our soldiers! Dr. Treva donates the candy to our deployed army men and women! So, we *did* talk about how we were sending candy to our soldiers. The kids made cards to send with their candy. What a rewarding way to give up something meaningful for the sake of others (and *their* cavities! Just kidding).

Blog Post—December—What My Kids Think

My husband had this great idea of letting our kids blog! I thought it might be nice for you to hear what *they* think of our New Years' Resolution of 2010...as the family members sort of forced to deal with it! Here's what our older children said, in their own words:

Liz (10) said:
"What!!!???
How could you go on without buying new things?
Well, going to parties and having to make my own presents is cool and it gives me a chance to be creative.
What I learned is that you don't have to buy things that are factory-made. You make the presents.
When a person receives a gift if it is home-made or hand-made by you it is more special because...they know that you spent time on their gift.
I also noticed that YES! It is hard. But it can make a difference in your life. You can think, *Wow! I made something.* You will be able to pay your bills faster and not have to worry about not having enough money to pay."

Here's what Matt (11) had to say:
"The experience of us only buying used stuff really helped me connect to God. The reason why is because God gave everything He had to us. He didn't go to a store and get it; He gave everything He had. So, I would inspire you to use what you have and use it wisely."
WOW! Even I was a little surprised by their responses! What a blessing to know that our kids got something out of this experience too!

Chapter 15

According to Our Kids

When I talk to other parents or read books or articles[1] on families raising children earth-consciously, I hear over and over again of the benefits for the kids. When kids live on less, or on what they already have, they learn that their happiness isn't about what they acquire or own. Happiness, then, has to come from other, healthier, more true places.

Kids learn that they can live within their means. They don't see debt or excessive buying modeled in their parents. They see and experience the possibility of living with what you have and enjoying it. They are less likely to utilize debt if they've been trained to save and live simply.

Kids learn that it's okay to be different. This is a toughie, and one that certainly pricked my heart for them early on. There's a number of reasons we're different: their grandmother was murdered by their grandfather (read our book *While We Slept: Finding Hope and Healing After Homicide*). They were raised in a blended family of foster siblings, adoptive siblings, and birth siblings (we've got books on this, too). They were raised in a multi-ethnic family with a white Californian mama and an African-Colombian-American daddy. They were raised in a family who pursues alternative care. And we went ahead and added not buying anything new and living with what we have. Most of the time. So being different isn't new. But it still pricks my heart when they go to a friend's house and see a room overflowing with toys and come home and ask, "Why don't we have that many toys?" So, we talk about the experiences we've shared. The twenty-five different countries they've been to by the ages (now) of eleven and twelve. Getting to learn languages and instruments. And we ask if they could trade those memories for a world full of toys, would they? And normally they say no. Now we're entering the years of devices, where some kids have phones and tablets and iPods and computers. And our kids will be different yet again.

They've learned generosity and short holds on things. In fact, they're often better at this than I am. My daughter can receive a birthday gift, love it well for a day, and be ready to pass it on. Internally, I'm like, *No! It's so cute! And the gift-giver will be so sad or offended! We should hang onto it until…*but then I remember my *why* for our wacko lifestyle. I don't want to reshape a beautiful gift of giving things away into a sentimental or obligatory hold on *stuff*. She's taught *me* to practice letting go.

I often find, in my own parenting, that one of my strongest desires is to protect them from pain. I want to shield them from everything hurtful. But knowing that kids *also* need to feel a sense of contribution to the world, an ability to be good at something, independence, and connection, I have to step out of the way (with guidance, of course). I don't mean at their detriment; I mean *for their growth*. Letting them feel the sting of being different released them to feel the joy of those differences. Letting them work through their own challenges released them to experience their own capability. Letting them make mistakes (ah!) released them to grow from the lessons of their failures, get comfortable with humility, and explore gratitude. The depth that comes from traversing hard things together (versus saving them from every possible pain) develops each of us. Preventing pain feels good in the short-term but raises kids with no depth…kind of like that puddle.

Not that a life of choosing to live conscientiously is full of pain. There's so much joy! And there's also so much rubbing against the culture, and the rub can make us raw. But I wouldn't trade the lessons we learn together, and that they'll take with them into their own homes and future, for anything else in the world. You can't put a dollar amount on security, maturity, and character borne in the fires of counter-cultural living.

Well, I suppose it would have been enough if we had done our year and called it good, returning back to our previous ways of spending and living. But come the end of the year, I suddenly had a new, brilliant inspiration for what we could do *next*. Read on to learn what 2011 had for us (and the ways it changed our forever in even bigger ways).

---

[1] Becker, J. (2010). How to Become Minimalist with Children. Retrieved May 23, 2020, from https://www.becomingminimalist.com/how-to-become-minimalist-with-children/

Blog Post—November—Countdown is On!

There are 32 days left in this year. Where has the time gone? It's rather amazing. I thought "old" people were strange when I was young and they would say, "Time passes more quickly the older you get!" I must be old. Time is passing by rather quickly. Far more so than it seemed to as a kid.

I remember it feeling excruciatingly long between Thanksgiving and Christmas. Now I hardly have a chance to catch my breath after the large turkey meal before we are making a *lot* of noise bringing in the New Year! What is this strange phenomenon that makes the same increments of time seem slower or faster depending on age? I'll save the answer to that mystery for another blog.

Back to the thirty-two days until the end of this year. I guess that means today marks the 333rd day of our 2010 resolution to not buy anything new. It's...shocking? That we made it this long? Not that I didn't expect to. I'm a very goal-oriented person and stick to my decisions (when I make them) very well. Others were skeptical. But here we are. We have failed a few times, both intentionally and accidentally. But the lessons we have gathered, the people we have met, the deeper relationship with God, are all such unexpected blessings to what we thought was just an experiment with the excess of our nation.

Someone asked recently if we've saved lots of money this year. It didn't seem so initially. I really like Neighborhood Thrift! But when I consider that we've had a pay cut this year due to the economy, like so many others, and that we adopted two children in the last year...the answer must be yes! It feels as though we are still paycheck to paycheck...and we are. But our paycheck is considerably less and we are still making it!

Will we continue this on into the new year? In so many ways, definitely. Will I have guilt and shame when I buy something "new"? No way! But I won't trade in the gift of seeing God provide for my own convenience anymore (hopefully!). Those riches have far outweighed my own ability to meet my own needs. How about you?

Chapter 16

New Challenge

2010 came to an end and we survived. No, we *thrived*. We dealt with our failures, wept over the gratitude of unexpected gifts, and were forever marked by our decision to only buy used. And suddenly, I had a new idea. Don't worry, you're near the end of the book! I can imagine the look on your face. "Oh my word, are we starting a whole new adventure?" HA! No, but I am going to leave you with this one.

I don't recall the exact moment it came to me, but undoubtedly it was the result of 2010. Having been so slow in our purchases, spent so much time on experiences as a family, and realizing how much *stuff* equals *sound* to me, I approached my family with a new idea.

What if we gave away half of our belongings in 2011?

Silence.

Well, except for my husband who was an immediate, "YES, I'm in." Having been raised between the countries of the United States and Colombia, and moving quite a bit therein, he was also accustomed to living on little. The death of his mom and following incarceration of his father suddenly took us from a minimalist apartment worth of things, to an entire house *and* apartment worth of things. Then we began fostering children, and with them came all sorts of regulations around what's required. Each child had to have a desk of their own (even if they worked at the table or on the couch). Each child had to have $50 of brand-new clothing *every month*. While they themselves often came with little, the regulations surrounding them brought a lot more stuff. Then we had babies. More stuff. Then, then, then. Even without buying new things for a whole year, we still had *too much*.

We talked it through as a family and finally came to an agreement. We would do it. This was before we had Marie Kondo showing us how to choose or organize this process of exterminating half of our belongings. We were on our own. No KonMari Method for us!

How do you even measure something like this? How do you know when you've hit half? Is it size? Actual items? Does a box of Littlest Pet Shop toys count as one or 500? Does a piano count as one or 500? We didn't know, so we made it up as we went. The words of Duane Elgin from 1940 echoed into my present as we began, "The intention of voluntary simplicity is not to dogmatically live with less. It's a more demanding intention of living with balance. This is a middle way that moves between the extremes of poverty and indulgence." I knew this would help us find balance and the result would be freedom. At the end of the day, it didn't matter how we measured, only that we sought balance and peace.

I started with the closet and felt so accomplished when, in the first two days, I freed of us half our clothes. *This will be easy-peasy,* I thought. Then I went through our bathroom cupboards. Not bad. Then I made my way to all my years of Disney stuffed animals. *Ouch* *I'll come back to those*, I thought. So, I made my way to the kitchen. THE KITCHEN. Basically, only the first few days were easy. After that, I had to wrestle with all of my sentimentality, all of my previous poverty and scarcity mentality and fears and *What if*s. It was far harder than I thought. Marie Kondo said, "Just because you dispose of something does not mean you give up past experiences or your identity." This was something I was forced to confront when engaging every object in my house. It was powerful. It was painful.

The irony, though, that brings me to the point of this chapter is that *only God knew why He inspired us to get rid of half our items.*

We ended up getting rid of 95% of what we owned.

By the end of 2011, we sold or gave away nearly everything and temporarily moved into a furnished rental. We decided to take an opportunity to move to Germany to work at a Christian international school. And we were only taking our luggage and a handful of boxes.

Ninety-five percent of our stuff. That's a lot of stuff.

In the months before we moved to Germany, in the summer of 2012, we stored our packed luggage for Germany and rented a van for a month. We traveled the United States, visiting multiple states from California to Ohio and back again along the southern route. The six of us had the bags on our back, the perfect preparation for moving to Germany with considerably less.

Once we arrived in Germany, we *only* had our luggage. Our boxes took months to come and held books (We got rid of over half our books but *books!*) Eight years later, we have replaced the emptiness of our walls and shelves with things locally, mostly used and repurposed, but still *stuff.*

And so, all of these years beyond 2010 and 2011, we find ourselves still on a journey of living on less, loving what we have, and supporting local artists. We still live on primarily second-hand items. We still create and experience. We still question each item that comes in and what will leave to make room. And we still fail.

I suppose this journey will never end, but this is what keeps us fully present. I suppose if we ever fully engage autopilot on this thing, we'd lose the gratitude and intentionality that anchors us to our original decisions to be different. Even back in 1940, Doris Janzen Longacre knew the challenge. "The trouble with simple living is that, though it can be joyful, rich, and creative, it isn't simple."

It's been said that "Maybe the life you've always wanted to live is buried underneath everything you own."

Then I'm going to keep digging and letting go. What about you?

Blog Post—January 2011—Last Day or First Day?

Merry Christmas! Or rather, Happy New Year! Today marks the end (or is it just the beginning? *wink*) of our 2010 New Year's Resolution. WE MADE IT!

I can't believe that an entire year has passed since this crazy idea spawned in my thoughts. It has been such a cool experience!

Over our Christmas holiday we visited family in Arizona. One individual was so interested in our resolution, he couldn't figure out what we would do if we had to buy new shoes during the year! It was kind of funny...but only because it made us realize that, in some respects, social class or upbringing can really frame your opinion of this endeavor. My husband and I come from two different backgrounds in this respect, and that has always been interesting. Anyway, this individual made the point that shoes are a matter of health and need to be appropriate for your foot. That's true. But I don't generally go through more than one pair of shoes in a year! Or even a couple of years! I suppose if your particular feet required specialized shoes, that would be considered consumable.

A number of things struck us during this experiment, some of which I'll list here.

1. Okay, how wealthy is our country? We have soooo much stuff that we have to rent mini houses to store it all? I don't know about your city, but we have a Derrel's mini storage on nearly every corner. There may be even more of them than Starbucks!

    Anyway, not only do we have so much stuff that we have to store it, but we have so much stuff that we can sell it a *second* time. It's not enough to sell our stuff once, we sell it multiple times: yard sales, thrift stores, consignments stores. My friends in various countries around the world would fall over with a heart attack if they knew how much stuff we have!

2. Letting God meet our needs was so cool! It was interesting to see what things *He* thought we needed. It was also a blessing to see Him give gifts, things that we secretly wanted, that He would provide in some form or another. It just reminded us how much He is our Father, and not just a distant, cold, unconcerned master. Rather, He shows Himself a personable, relational, loving Dad who *loves* to give good things to His children. What a warm truth to rest in!

   Clarification: We also definitely believe God distributes money and uses that, in many respects, as a way of meeting our needs. It was just fascinating to see Him do it in His time and His way as opposed to us just running to Walmart to meet our own needs.

3. We met so many cool people! Conversations occurred that never would have if we'd just gone our own private way. We also discovered many gems of thrift stores in town. My favorite, of course, is Neighborhood Thrift. Not only do they run a really great operation, but they seriously work to serve the community and make things available to lower income families, both through job opportunities and affordable items. I love the mission behind that store.

4. Our kids, each at such crucial ages, picked up such valuable insights throughout the year. We had an amazing Christmas, even though many of their gifts (the ones from us) were "second hand." (You'd be surprised at how many gifts I found for them *brand new in boxes* but at thrift stores! That was always exciting.

So many other things learned and experienced that we are still processing and will share as we formulate their significance in our lives.

Will we do it again this year? Yes and no. It won't be a formal "New Year's Resolution" but we will definitely continue to buy as little as we can new. Why not? We gleaned such wonderful things! On the other hand, I won't feel guilty for buying something new if I just can't find it used. (Like a snow sled, which may end up being my first purchase!) Regardless, we hope that as you've journeyed this with us, that you have been inspired in some form to consider "things" for what they are, the great wealth of our nation, and the ways that we can help to conserve and give back.

Chapter 17

Your Turn

What about you?

What will you do with your life?

Our journey doesn't have to be *your* journey. But I hope you're on *a* journey.

Your journey to happiness, well-being, and a better planet may not come by choosing to buy used or get rid of half your things (though that would certainly get you started!) Yours might begin with supporting a cause you believe in, giving up your month of Starbucks and building schools in impoverished areas instead. It might be planting trees or community gardens. It might be in feeding homeless or working on public policy to improve quality of life situations for various people groups.

And my point isn't to say that whatever you do, you should do it without fear or failing or insecurity. Those will be partners along the way. But choose hope. Choose hope over fear and see what doors open in front of you. Watch chains fall away from a life that's held you down with anxiety, depression, and doubt. Choose hope.

I want you to taste the gratitude and joy of only owning what you need and loving what you own. You can do all the things and still totally miss it if its rooted in a resentful spirit. Engage the opportunity to build community and see yourself bloom. Blooming can feel scary. It's different. Uncomfortable. It's a stretching of stiff parts. It's a vulnerability to the sun above and the elements around. But blooming is beautiful, and it's evident to everyone around. A person blooming is a beautiful person.

I assure you, though, that if you are willing to step into a year like the one that challenged us, and meet it with all you've got, willing to change and be changed, you will experience gifts beyond what you can imagine. My most terrified *yeses* have birthed the most incredible life pivots.

I hope you won't close this book feeling vicariously refreshed through our experience, then do nothing to start your own. Refuse to spend another day wishing you had less clutter screaming at you or begrudging the world around you for being so frivolous and consumer-driven. Take action! Start today with *one thing*.

Try a new way. Meet some new people along the way. Find community. Find yourself. Find the *gift* of yourself.

Choose hope. Choose you. Choose the world.

You're not alone.

About Marcy Pusey

Marcy Pusey is the wife of an artist and the mother of four, but she's also tossed pizzas for a pizzeria, acted and sang in a musical, advocated for families with special needs, made appearances in a few movies, and mimed with balloon animals at the Halifax Busker Festival.

Marcy is also a Certified Rehabilitation Counselor and Certified Trauma and Resilience Practitioner, speaker, coach, and the best-selling author of books for adults and for children. She does her best writing on retreats with a nearby hot-tub, in any castle, within view of the sea, or in her cozy home in the Black Forest of Germany. Marcy loves the smiles and giggles of kids who see themselves in her pages and the tearful nods of adults who realize they're not alone by her words.

Marcy is the best-selling author of *Reclaiming Hope: Overcoming the Challenges of Parenting Foster and Adopted Children*, *Parenting Children of Trauma: The Foster-Adoption Guide to Understanding Attachment Disorder*, *While We Slept: Finding Hope and Healing After Homicide* for adults, and *Tercules*, *Weirdo and Willy*, *According to Corban*, *Bath Time Magic*, and *Speranza's Sweater* for children.

Watch her TEDx talks and learn more about her work, writing, and other resources at www.marcypusey.com.

Don't forget to grab your
Abundance of Less Action Guide Free!

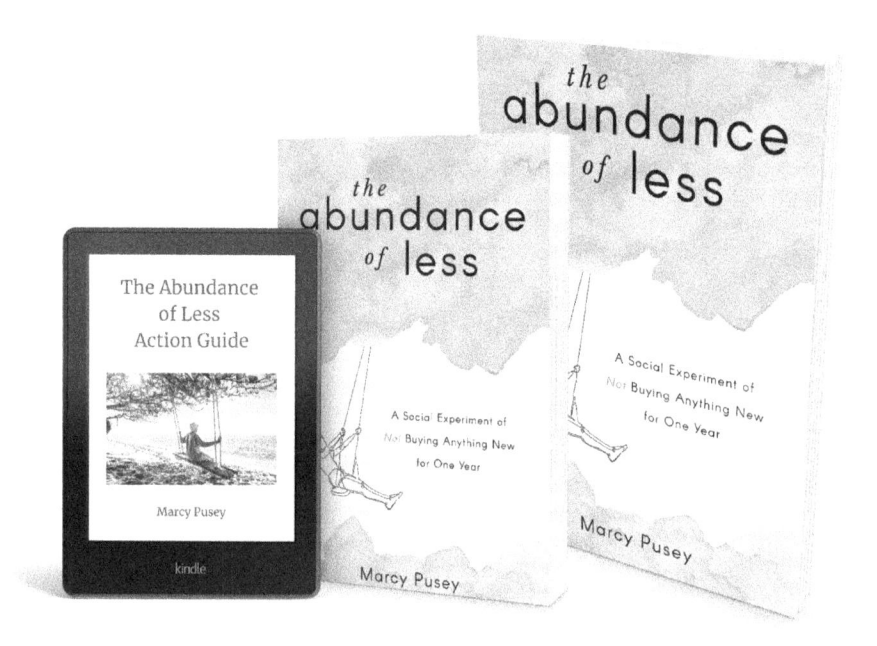

As a gift to help you get the most out of this book, we are giving you strategies, tips, and plans to help you execute your own year of living the abundance of less experience.

Download your free Action Guide at:

marcypusey.com/abundance-guide

Thank you for downloading my book!

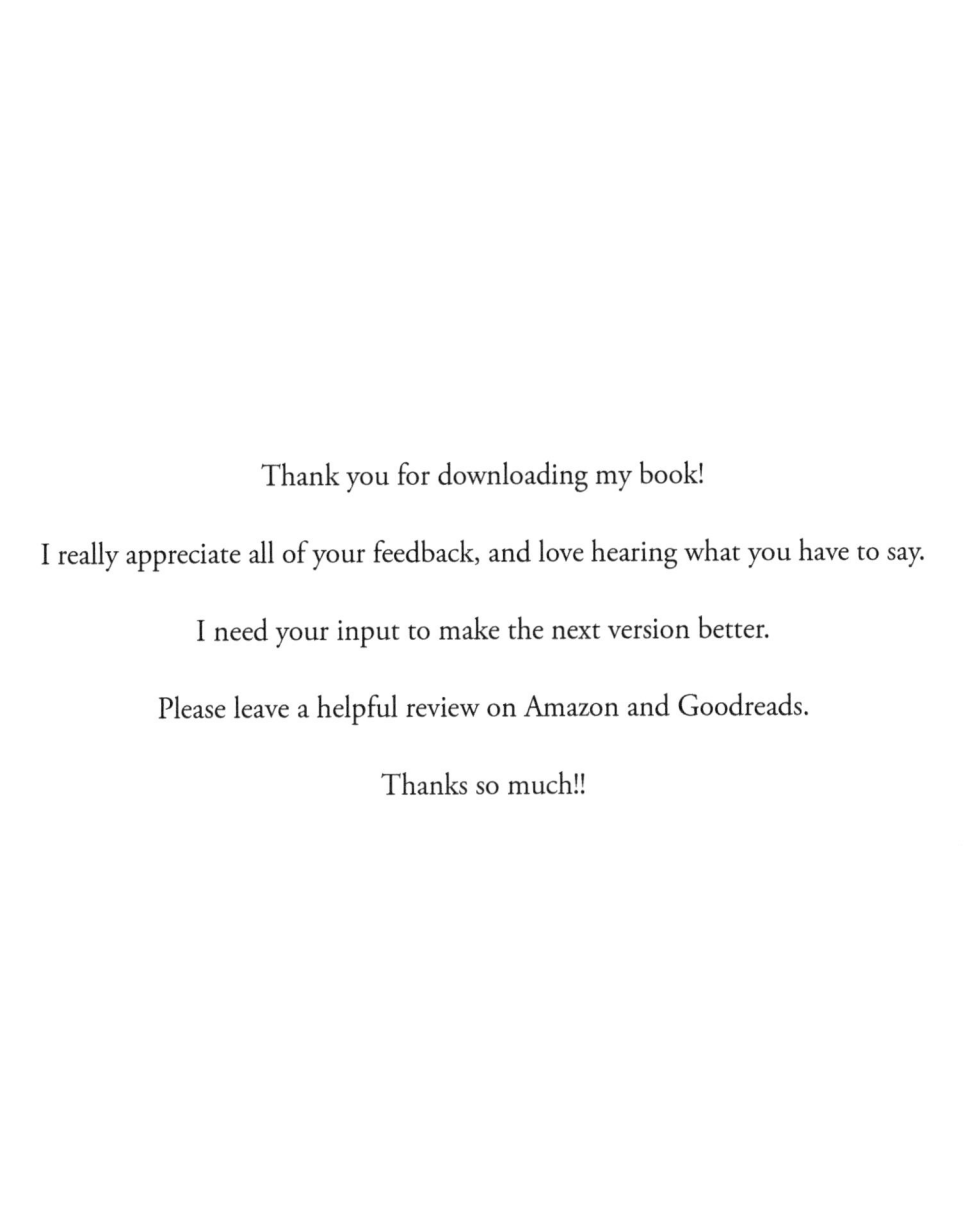

I really appreciate all of your feedback, and love hearing what you have to say.

I need your input to make the next version better.

Please leave a helpful review on Amazon and Goodreads.

Thanks so much!!

www.ingramcontent.com/pod-product-compliance
Ingram Content Group UK Ltd.
Pitfield, Milton Keynes, MK11 3LW, UK
UKHW041553300125
4377UKWH00022B/229